Mordecai Arieli

The Occupational Experience of Residential Child and Youth Care Workers: Caring and Its Discontents

Pre-publication
REVIEWS,
COMMENTARIES,
EVALUATIONS . . .

"**W**orks on care tend to be prescriptive: Most of them discuss what ought to be done with those in need of care–rather than describe what the reality of care actually looks like. Arieli's highly original book differs from so many others on this theme in precisely this aspect: it both describes reality, and analyses and examines theoretical issues. It refrains from setting rules and does not give advice as to how to better care for children and adolescents. But this apparently "non-practical" approach works well. It convinces me of the truth in Kurt Lewin's suggestion there is nothing more practical than a sound theory."

Gerald Mars, PhD
Professor
Management Centre
University of Bradford, England

"**M**ordecai Arieli sees the youth care worker mainly as a person who achieves self actualization through interaction with the youth in care and commitment toward their growth. Evidently, Arieli's main source of inspiration is the thinking of philosophers, sociologists, social psychologists and pedagogues of the symbolic interactionist school. Arieli refutes the notion that there are clear answers that can give the youth care workers a sense of certainty and security in their work. He emphasizes the constant state of questioning in adult-youth relations. Nevertheless, it appears that the message contained in Arieli's approach may be more effective in the training of youth care workers than an unequivocal message or prescription."

Dr. Simcha Shlasky
Lecturer
Sociology of Education
and Child Care
Center for Technological
Education
Holon, Israel

"**T**he literature dealing with youth care workers generally discusses their attitudes towards their charges or towards various aspects of their role in the residential organization, Mordecai Arieli adopts a different approach in his book. *The Occupational Experience of Residential Child and Youth Care Workers: Caring and Its Discontents* does not restrict the individual worker to expressing attitudes in one particular sphere or relate to him/her as someone filling an organizational role with a standard definition. Instead, the book documents the dynamic interaction between the worker and his/her charges, relating to the totality of the worker as a person. He or she is not an anonymous individual, one subject among many in a sample, but a person with his/her own identity and personal approach to work and to the surrounding world.

While contributing to academic research, this book fills an important didactic function. It is both a highly original ethnographic study of the world of youth care workers and a vital instrument for their training."

Yitzhak Kashti
Associate Professor
Tel-Aviv University
School of Education
Tel-Aviv, Israel

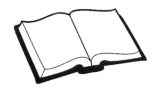
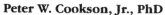

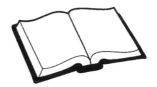

The Haworth Press, Inc.

The Occupational Experience of Residential Child and Youth Care Workers: Caring and Its Discontents

The Occupational Experience
of Residential Child
and Youth Care Workers:
Caring and Its Discontents

Mordecai Arieli

The Haworth Press, Inc.
New York • London

The Occupational Experience of Residential Child and Youth Care Workers: Caring and Its Discontents has also been published as *Child & Youth Services*, Volume 18, Number 2 1997.

The development, preparation, and publication of this work has been undertaken with great care. However, the publisher, employees, editors, and agents of The Haworth Press and all imprints of The Haworth Press, Inc., including The Haworth Medical Press and Pharmaceutical Products Press, are not responsible for any errors contained herein or for consequences that may ensue from use of materials or information contained in this work. Opinions expressed by the author(s) are not necessarily those of The Haworth Press, Inc.

Cover design by Thomas J. Mayshock, Jr.

The Haworth Press, Inc., 10 Alice Street, Binghamton, NY 13904-1580 USA

Library of Congress Cataloging-in-Publication Data

Arieli, Mordecai.
    The occupational experience of residential child and youth care workers : caring and its discontents / Mordecai Arieli.
        p.   cm.
    Also published as Child & youth services, vol. 18, no. 2, 1997.
    Includes bibliographical references and index.
    ISBN 1-56024-784-3 (alk. paper).–ISBN 0-7890-0306-6 (pbk. : alk. paper)
        1. Children–Institutional care–Great Britain. 2. Child care workers–Great Britain. I. Title.
HV866.G7A75 1997   97-7841
362.73′2′0941–dc21   CIP

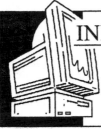

INDEXING & ABSTRACTING

Contributions to this publication are selectively indexed or abstracted in print, electronic, online, or CD-ROM version(s) of the reference tools and information services listed below. This list is current as of the copyright date of this publication. See the end of this section for additional notes.

- *Cambridge Scientific Abstracts*, *Risk Abstracts*, Environmental Routenet (accessed via INTERNET), 7200 Wisconsin Ave #601, Bethesda, MD 20814

- *Child Development Abstracts & Bibliography*, University of Kansas, 2 Bailey Hall, Lawrence, KS 66045

- *CNPIEC Reference Guide: Chinese National Directory of Foreign Periodicals* P.O. Box 88, Beijing, Peoples Republic of China

- *Criminal Justice Abstracts*, Willow Tree Press, 15 Washington Street, 4th Floor, Newark, NJ 07102

- *Criminology, Penology and Police Science Abstracts*, Kugler Publications, P. O. Box 11188, 1001 GD Amsterdam, The Netherlands

- *ERIC Clearinghouse on Counseling and Student Services (ERIC/CASS)*, University of North Carolina-Greensboro, 101 Park Building, Greensboro, NC 27412-5001

- *ERIC Clearinghouse on Elementary & Early Childhood Education*, University of Illinois, 805 West Pennsylvania Avenue, Urbana, IL 61801

- *Exceptional Child Education Resources (ECER), (CD/ROM from SilverPlatter and hard copy)*, The Council for Exceptional Children, 1920 Association Drive, Reston, VA 22091

- *Family Studies Database (online and CD/ROM)*, National Information Services Corporation, 306 East Baltimore Pike, 2nd Floor, Media, PA 19063

- *IBZ International Bibliography of Periodical Literature*, Zeller Verlag GmbH & Co., P.O.B. 1949, d-49009 Osnabruck, Germany

- *Index to Periodical Articles Related to Law*, University of Texas, 727 East 26th Street, Austin, TX 78705

- *International Bulletin of Bibliography on Education*, Proyecto B.I.B.E./Apartado 52, San Lorenzo del Escorial, Madrid, Spain

(continued)

- *INTERNET ACCESS (& additional networks) Bulletin Board for Libraries ("BUBL"), coverage of information resources on INTERNET, JANET, and other networks.*
  - JANET X.29: UK.AC.BATH.BUBL or 00006012101300
  - TELNET: BUBL.BATH.AC.UK or 138.38.32.45 login 'bubl'
  - Gopher: BUBL.BATH.AC.UK (138.32.32.45). Port 7070
  - World Wide Web: http: / / www.bubl.bath.ac.uk./BUBL/ home.html
  - NISSWAIS: telnetniss.ac.uk (for the NISS gateway)
  The Andersonian Library, Curran Building, 101 St. James Road, Glasgow G4 ONS, Scotland

- *Mental Health Abstracts (online through DIALOG)*, IFI/Plenum Data Company, 3202 Kirkwood Highway, Wilmington, DE 19808

- *OT BibSys, American Occupational Therapy Foundation*, P. O. Box 31220, Rockville, MD 20824-1220

- *PASCAL International Bibliography T205: Sciences de l'information Documentation*, INIST/CNRS-Service Gestion des Documents Primaires, 2, allee du Parc de Brabois, F-54514 Vandoeuvre-les-Nancy, Cedex, France

- *Psychological Abstracts (PsycINFO)*, American Psychological Association, P. O. Box 91600, Washington, DC 20090-1600

- *Referativnyi Zhurnal (Abstracts Journal of the Institute of Scientific Information of the Republic of Russia)*, The Institute of Scientific Information, Baltijskaja ul., 14, Moscow A-219, Republic of Russia

- *Sage Family Studies Abstracts*, Sage Publications, Inc., 2455 Teller Road, Newbury Park, CA 91320

- *Social Planning/Policy & Development Abstracts (SOPODA)*, Sociological Abstracts, Inc., P. O. Box 22206, San Diego, CA 92192-0206

- *Social Work Abstracts*, National Association of Social Workers, 750 First Street NW, 8th Floor, Washington, DC 20002

- *Sociological Abstracts (SA)*, Sociological Abstracts, Inc., P. O. Box 22206, San Diego, CA 92192-0206

- *Sociology of Education Abstracts*, Carfax Publishing Company, P. O. Box 25, Abingdon, Oxfordshire OX14 3UE, United Kingdom

- *Studies on Women Abstracts*, Carfax Publishing Company, P. O. Box 25, Abingdon, Oxfordshire OX14 3UE, United Kingdom

- *Violence and Abuse Abstracts: A Review of Current Literature on Interpersonal Violence (VAA)*, Sage Publications, Inc., 2455 Teller Road, Newbury Park, CA 91320

(continued)

SPECIAL BIBLIOGRAPHIC NOTES

related to special journal issues (separates)
and indexing/abstracting

☐ indexing/abstracting services in this list will also cover material in any "separate" that is co-published simultaneously with Haworth's special thematic journal issue or DocuSerial. Indexing/abstracting usually covers material at the article/chapter level.

☐ monographic co-editions are intended for either non-subscribers or libraries which intend to purchase a second copy for their circulating collections.

☐ monographic co-editions are reported to all jobbers/wholesalers/approval plans. The source journal is listed as the "series" to assist the prevention of duplicate purchasing in the same manner utilized for books-in-series.

☐ to facilitate user/access services all indexing/abstracting services are encouraged to utilize the co-indexing entry note indicated at the bottom of the first page of each article/chapter/contribution.

☐ this is intended to assist a library user of any reference tool (whether print, electronic, online, or CD-ROM) to locate the monographic version if the library has purchased this version but not a subscription to the source journal.

☐ individual articles/chapters in any Haworth publication are also available through the Haworth Document Delivery Services (HDDS).

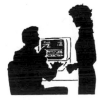

The Occupational Experience of Residential Child and Youth Care Workers: Caring and Its Discontents

CONTENTS

And all the while, close behind him stood Mrs. Bedoneby-asyoudid.

Some people may say: But why did she not keep her cupboard locked? Well, I know. It seems a very strange thing, but she never does keep her cupboard locked; every one may go and taste for themselves, and fare accordingly. It is very odd, but so it is; and I am quite sure that she knows best. Perhaps she wishes people to keep their fingers out of the fire, by having them burnt. She took off her spectacles, because she did not like to see too much, and in her pity she arched up her eyebrows into her very hair, and her eyes grew so wide that they would have taken in all the sorrow of the world, and filled with great big tears as they often do. But all she said was "Ah, You poor little dear! You are just like all the rest."

. . . But what did the strange fairy do when she saw all her lollipops eaten?

Did she fly at Tom, catch him by the scruff of the neck, hold him, howk him, hump him, hurry him, hit him, poke him, pull him, pinch him, pound him, put him in the corner, shake him, slap him, set him on a cold stone to reconsider himself, and so forth?

Not a bit . . . You will never see her do that. For, if she had, she knew quite well, Tom would have fought, and kicked, and bit, and said bad words, and turned again that moment into a naughty little heathen chimney sweep, with his hands, like Ishmael of old, against every man, and every man against him.

. . . No. She leaves that for anxious parents and teachers (lazy ones, some call them), who, instead of giving children a fair trial, force them by fright to confess their own faults—which is so cruel and unfair that no judge on the bench dare do it to the wickedest thief or murderer, for the good British law forbids it. . . . It is never committed now, save by Inquisitors, and Kings of Naples, and a few other wretched people of whom the world is weary.

Charles Kingsley, *The Water-Babies* 1863

ABOUT THE AUTHOR

Mordecai Arieli, PhD, is a sociologist of educational organizations who specializes in sociology of residential schools and childcare facilities and interaction between children and adults. He has been a faculty member of the Tel-Aviv University School of Education since 1975. At the University, he has served as Head of the following departments and programs: Educational Administration, Teacher Training in the Social Sciences, Research in the Sociology of Education and the Community In-service Training of Teachers and Principals, and the Training of Residential-Education Staff. Dr Arieli has been an influential advisor to many Israeli residential education programs, including Israel's leading agency in the field, Youth Aliyah. The author of *Residential Schools: Staffs and Communities* and *Teaching and Its Discontents* and the co-author of *Residential Schools as People-Processing Organizations* and *The Residential Education Alternative*, his major areas of interest include role perceptions, interaction, and conflicts of residential staff and inmates.

Foreword

When the headmaster of Westminster School, a boarding institution of some antiquity, numbering as it does several Saxon Kings among its alumni, foresees the closure of its dormitories within several years, then decay is in the air. The loss of "Happyhours" small group home hardly robs the national heritage, but the prospect of long grass growing in the courts of Eton and Winchester or of Sherborne's cloister as host to McDonald's and Carpetland causes some to be concerned. For others, the decline excites nostalgia, for most quiet euphoria.

Residence for children and young people is in decline, particularly in educational and welfare contexts. However, the shrinkage is more marked in some sectors of provision than others. In 1971 a reliable estimate showed that in the United Kingdom 300,000 young people sat down to an institutional breakfast; by 1991 that number of children, eighteen years and younger, had fallen to about 200,000. Some groups have diminished dramatically, particularly children in long-stay hospitals and those in state care.

The impetus began in the early 1970s with the closure of the reformatories, unlovely survivors from the nineteenth century industrial and reformatory schools. In 1971 they sheltered about 8,000 boys and 1,000 girls under the age of eighteen; today less than 800 are away from home at such places. Small group homes that accommodated children in state care followed; in 1971 they held 41,000 children; by 1991, 12,000; and today the number hovers around 8,000. During the 1980s the special boarding schools for children with behavioral and emotional difficulties shared the exodus. In 1971, those with physical or mental disabilities in residential settings numbered 35,000; by 1991 they had dwindled to 19,000.

Neither is the decline in the use of residential care confined to vulnerable, disadvantaged, and disruptive young people. Our prestigious boarding schools, of which Westminster School is one, have also suffered. Numbers have fallen from 141,000 in 1971 to 103,000 by 1991 and the

[Haworth co-indexing entry note]: "Foreword," Millham, Spencer. Co-published simultaneously in *Child & Youth Services* (The Haworth Press, Inc.) Vol. 18, No. 2, 1997, pp. xv-xviii; and: *The Occupational Experience of Residential Child and Youth Care Workers: Caring and Its Discontents* (Mordecai Arieli) The Haworth Press, Inc., 1997, pp. xv-xviii. Single or multiple copies of this article are available for a fee from The Haworth Document Delivery Service [1-800-342-9678, 9:00 a.m. - 5:00 p.m. (EST). E-mail address: getinfo@haworth.com].

decline is accelerating. Here a delay in the age at which children start boarding has been a major factor.

These figures, if anything, conceal even more changes in the residential care of children. The move in state care has not been towards alternative provision such as foster care but to keeping children at home. This is particularly true with younger children and is echoed in the education sector where special needs are met in the local day schools. Unfortunately, the improvements in day and local community provision for children and families have meant that in state care those who end up in residence are hard to place, problematic adolescents. Indeed, the only residential sector that has shown remarkable resilience over the decades provides highly specialized treatment and/or maximum security, which has grown from 350 places in 1971 to about 500 places in 1991 and is still growing. In penal provision, there has been polarization, with far fewer younger boys removed from home but less reduction among those of sixteen years and older.

In state residential provision, the move has been to more short-term, crisis, needs-led services, much more flexibility in style, location, and size, and closer integration with other social, health, and educational services. In the independent boarding schools, there has been a marked drop in numbers of younger residents, more weekly or termly boarders, that is, short-term boarding, and much more flexibility in provision. Attempts to check the drift home by co-education and recruitment abroad have only been partly successful.

What is noticeable in all provisions with the exception of maximum security is the increasing voice of children in where they go and what they receive linked with much greater awareness and participation of parents, particularly mothers, in making a choice.

How far decline and change in the UK's residential sector characterizes other countries is difficult to estimate. Comparisons between sectors of care and categories of children are complicated and many countries do not gather relevant data. Obviously, these changes are very significant in the UK and are shared by others in the European Community: France, Italy, and Germany. In the USA, in many states, the residential sector is resilient because of increasingly punitive attitudes to young delinquents and rapid growth in the numbers of young people separated in state care.

In Israel, where the following study was done, residential care is also in slow decline. High numbers of children linger in institutional care in erstwhile communist countries not because such is prized but because alternatives are slow to develop. Generally, it is difficult to get an accurate picture because the relationship between care, special needs, educational, and "elite," sectors of residential care differ across societies.

Nevertheless, the following scrutiny of the staff world of residential institutions is very opportune. Usually concerns with adaptations and outcomes for children elbow aside much consideration of staff, their reasons for seeking employment in residential work, their aspirations and experience. In the UK, the declining and changing role of residence has had a marked effect upon staff morale and recruitment. Limited career structures have shrunk while training and expertise encourage staff to leave for wider social or educational employment.

Residential care institutions usually employ more women than men, often attracting those attempting a second career and those whose aspirations are in excess of their qualifications. Hence, training and appropriate professional support are at a premium, particularly as the children are difficult. In the UK residential staff in child care do not stay long, they either burn out or drop out, and there is little reward for a long stay, as the residential homes are difficult to change and improve. Wider changes in the labor market have also had an effect, unionization has increased the labor costs of care, and the expansion of women's employment, slow increases in their pay, and the flexibility of part-time employment have all discouraged a career in residential care.

This crisis in the staff world of residential institutions is not so marked in the independent boarding schools; staff are usually highly qualified and can move either between schools or into wider education. Nevertheless, those seeking a boarding role have diminished and ancillary care staff are in short supply.

This insecurity can express itself in staff feelings of discontent, as Mordecai Arieli indicates in the following pages. Such discontent may also spring from the meanings that staff members impute to young people's responses in daily interactions. In any case, staff certainly cannot take youthful cooperation for granted.

If anything, insecurity and financial pressures are stronger on boarding schools; although they have long sheltered children who need boarding for family reasons, the schools are in business and the decline in sales has led to many closures. The schools are also vulnerable to political change, as one third of their places are "assisted," attracting considerable state subsidy and they uneasily enjoy the considerable tax benefits of "charity" status. This could easily change.

To those of us with long memories who shivered in the gaunt halls of the reformatory schools in the 1960s or shuffled uneasily as boys sang morning hymns beneath the wonderful ceilings and asphyxiating glass of awesome school chapels, this crisis is depressingly familiar. There is a belated chorus of how valuable a national resource residential care represents, a flurry of committees, even a research programme. High sounding phrases abound, such as residential care providing a seamless web of services, or a "needs-led resource."

Although the rhetoric changes, the truth does not. Residential care needs highly qualified staff, professional support, attractive career structures, and good working conditions. It needs to be esteemed. Unfortunately, such conditions in both state care and in our independent boarding schools price their provision out of the market. Costly, inward-looking, and resistant to change, prone to scandal and difficult to manage, nobody wants to run them.

Of course, it is a long way from our crumbling, mock Gothic facades to the youth villages and kibbutzim of Israel. Although the functions of residential care may have changed in recent years, there boarding may still have a rosy future. In many Israeli residential schools Rachel may still provocatively pick avocados in the sunshine, earning enough to take her to the Sabbath discos of Tel Aviv. Not quite the residential style the headmaster of Westminster had in mind as he bewailed the decline of our schools. But I know where I would rather be!

Spencer Millham
Dartington Social Research Unit
University of Bristol, UK

Preface

Twice in my professional career I have experienced the pleasure and the honor of meeting Professor Mordecai Arieli–once in Switzerland at a meeting of the International Federation of Educative Communities (FICE), and once in Israel, while I was attending a special FICE seminar on training and education in child and youth work. These experiences are sustained with the special opportunity I have to write the preface of *The Occupational Experience of Residential Child and Youth Care Workers: Caring and Its Discontents*.

Today we are at a crossroads in residential child and youth care work. While the youth that primary child and youth care workers are called upon to serve are increasingly disturbed often in multiple aspects of their functioning working conditions are becoming more difficult and the availability of needed resources and other supports for the work is decreasing. It is important that we truly recognize the impact of these on the workers who comprise the field if we wish to continue to move it forward as an essential human service. Paradoxically, this very situation offers a mandate to do so, and certainly knowing more about the core nature of the work–both its "discontents" and "contents"–is crucial to the effort. *The Occupational Experience of Residential Child and Youth Care Workers: Caring and Its Discontents* offers a unique and timely perspective on these significant aspects and encourages us to take the road forward.

Occupational discontent in the field has previously been addressed by authors and researchers who have chosen other focal points around which to frame their studies, such as burnout and stress, turnover and retention, salaries, and overall working conditions. This is important information, of course. But when combined with real, qualitative data about the nature of daily experience with youth such as offered here, it has much more utility.

Thus a major contribution of this volume is providing child and youth care workers themselves an open voice–indeed, permission to speak honestly– which yields the acknowledgment that there are elements of discontent in

[Haworth co-indexing entry note]: "Preface," VanderVen, Karen. Co-published simultaneously in *Child & Youth Services* (The Haworth Press, Inc.) Vol. 18, No. 2, 1997, pp. xix-xxi; and: *The Occupational Experience of Residential Child and Youth Care Workers: Caring and Its Discontents* (Mordecai Arieli) The Haworth Press, Inc., 1997, pp. xix-xxi. Single or multiple copies of this article are available for a fee from The Haworth Document Delivery Service [1-800-342-9678, 9:00 a.m. - 5:00 p.m. (EST). E-mail address: getinfo@haworth.com].

the work above and beyond the structural factors just cited. Making such process information manifest is crucial in providing us the kind of insights we need in order to help the field advance into a full profession and to select and focus our activities so as to address the real dynamics that hinder such progress. This book effectively bridges both naive idealism about how wonderful it is to "work with people," as in child and youth work, and the paralyzing depression about how it is impossible to improve the situation of the disenchanted worker, both of which have impeded the field in the past.

The constructivist approach of *The Occupational Experience of Residential Child and Youth Care Workers: Caring and Its Discontents* is focused on the culture that situates caring interactions and on the perceived experience of the caregivers. This is highly congruent with contemporary methodological trends in psychology and human development, which are oriented toward producing new knowledge that is highly based in social experience, its cultural context, and the meaning that people make of that experience. And if, as is often contended, the interactions with youth are the crux of the developmental work we do with them, then this work not only provides a window into the significance of interactions, but also illuminates their actual characteristics. Such veracity is essential if we are to truly legitimize this core function of the field in the future.

The Occupational Experience of Residential Child and Youth Care Workers: Caring and Its Discontents gives me great optimism for the field of caring. Why? One might say, "This is so pessimistic. Look at how difficult and unrewarding caring is." Not at all. First of all, the volume demystifies the work. It openly speaks about things we have not talked about, although their presence has always been both implicit and explicit, such as issues of power and control. Secondly, we must bear in mind that *any* of life's endeavors have unpleasant aspects—certainly work does, even where members of the occupation love and are committed to it, as are many of those who participated in Professor Arieli's study. If we are serious in our efforts to define, conceptualize, and advance the field or profession of primary caregiving, then this is exactly the kind of source information we need. The volume also offers supporting and new perspectives on other key areas of caring work, such as values, training and education, and practitioner roles.

I have stated in my own writing that "control" is a major value underlying many approaches to dealing with difficult youth in out-of-home services. This is confirmed in this work, but in a way that has implications for truly understanding the dynamics of control and hence designing positive interventions rather than ones that simply serve to increase out-of-control behavior without therapeutic benefit.

Committed to the cruciality of rich activity programming as a core therapeutic and developmental intervention for children and youth, I found support for this in the fact that the workers in this study identified "idleness" as a major interference in their work, and boredom was a frequent youth complaint. These finding should serve as a "wake-up" call to us all to bring activity programming, often a neglected area, to the fore, both in practice and in refining the functions of the field.

As it is increasingly recognized that training and education are the linchpin for advancement of the field into professional effectiveness, the findings of *The Occupational Experience of Residential Child and Youth Care Workers: Caring and Its Discontents* hold particular significance, for they truly provide direct insight into the "texture" of the work. Supported by comments from the workers that contentment can increase with appropriate training, this study can be a rich source of target domains for curricular initiatives and innovation.

In his own comments about the purpose of the work, Professor Arieli describes the positions he has held for almost 40 years as a direct worker, a teacher, a supervisor, a trainer and educator, and a researcher, and he acknowledges that his own memories of discontent in his earlier working days are still vivid.

We are all fortunate that despite these experiences, he found a way to remain in the field and to do this study, which offers us so much substantive insight into the "psychosocial interior" of the working life of the child and youth care worker. In fact, this comment as well as the entire work reinforce my constant contention that we must support the creation and sustainment of multiple role options in the field in order for it to advance. Mobility among roles increases retention and provides a lifelong committed workforce.

I obviously have found much richness, enlightenment and confirmation in *The Occupational Experience of Residential Child and Youth Care Workers: Caring and Its Discontents*. Other readers will find in it similar areas and ideas to confirm, challenge, or stimulate their thinking.

I hope this seminal work will be widely read and utilized in the much needed task for our field of conceptualizing its function and knowledge base, confirming and further describing the domains of competency that workers need to develop for successful practice, and designing effective training and delivery systems.

Discontent can serve as an energizer. Let us use *The Occupational Experience of Residential Child and Youth Care Workers: Caring and Its Discontents* as an impetus to address these tasks in the immediate future.

Karen VanderVen
Professor and Program Director
Program in Child Development and Child Care
University of Pittsburgh

Acknowledgments

This work, its preparation and writing, were directly inspired by the works of many pedagogues and scholars in residential child care and education. Among these are some who have consistently influenced this and other work of mine in these fields. I wish to thank the dead and the living for the part they played in shaping my thinking on the world of residential care workers.

I learned much from Dr. Ovadia Aviram, Professor Moshe Smilansky, and Professor Martin Wolins.

I am grateful to Professor Haim Adlor, Professor Roger Bullock, Professor Rouven Feuerstein, Meir Gottesman, Professor Reuven Kahane, Dr. Mike Little, Professor Spencer Millham, and Esti Ray (my research assistant).

Special thanks for the fascinating and constructive discussions on the world of carers or other relevant issues of human interaction are due to the following: Professor Jerry Beker, Abigail Bracha, Professor Julius Carlebach, Nivi Gal, Professor Yitzhak Kashti, Daniella Kelem, Zvi Levy, Professor Rina Shapira, and Dr. Simcha Shlasky. I also wish to thank Hazel Arieli, whose linguistic sensitivity and watchful eye miss almost nothing, and the Israel Pollak Unit of Sociology of Education and the Community at the Tel Aviv University School of Education for funding the research on which this volume is based.

Introduction:
A Guiding Approach

— The residential care setting brings a world of children or adolescents together with a world of adults, often one adult acting alone–the group care worker. It also brings a world of those who are considered, for one reason or another, "not properly socialized"–whom the prevalent educational and care approaches seek to change–together with a world of those who know the "proper" social codes and are expected to generate the desired change in the ones who don't by intervening in the course of their maturation.

Thus, no matter how liberal they are, residential settings and their staffs intervene in their charges' maturation process. This results from the goals of the residential setting and the nature of the people acting in it: adults vis-à-vis youth, group care workers vis-à-vis those under their care. This intervention leads the youth to regard the group care worker as a somewhat coercive figure. In these circumstances, the youth often resist or seek to limit the group care worker's intervention.

This situation is not the function of a specific culture or residential setting and the method of care practiced in it, but results largely from the coercive intervention of socializing action. Group care workers tend to channel their charges into processes of change that are often stressful. Consequently, the group care worker is liable to be an unpopular figure, and his or her interaction with the youth sometimes teeters on the verge of crisis. The group care worker's experience of being on the verge of crisis disrupts the work and leads to a feeling which will be described here as discontent.

In this volume I will try to clarify some aspects of this phenomenon with the help of ethnographic interviews with group care workers in one

[Haworth co-indexing entry note]: "Introduction: A Guiding Approach." Arieli, Mordecai. Co-published simultaneously in *Child & Youth Services* (The Haworth Press, Inc.) Vol. 18, No. 2, 1997, pp. 1-10; and: *The Occupational Experience of Residential Child and Youth Care Workers: Caring and Its Discontents* (Mordecai Arieli) The Haworth Press, Inc., 1997, pp. 1-10. Single or multiple copies of this article are available for a fee from The Haworth Document Delivery Service [1-800-342-9678, 9:00 a.m. - 5:00 p.m. (EST). E-mail address: getinfo@haworth.com].

1

country, Israel, arguing that the ethnographic material presented transcends the boundaries of any one culture or situation.

THE CRUCIAL QUESTIONS

In what circumstances do group care workers perceive their role as associated with discontent? What are the sources of this discontent? Who causes them to feel discontent, why, how, and in what situations? Can they define the characteristics of the group care worker who feels particularly discontented? How do they cope with situations of discontent? How do they control the circumstances of caregiving situations so as to reduce the experience of discontent? In what respect and in what circumstances do the group care workers report that they find some contentment in their work?

At the beginning of this century, the German poet Rainer Maria Rilke advised a young poet who was reflecting upon his future path as follows: "Now live the questions, and then possibly one day, without even noticing it, you will be living into the answer." In the spirit of Rilke's advice, this book will discuss a problem in the world of group care workers without offering complete answers.

PURPOSE

In the course of the study that served as the basis for this volume, group care workers spoke about the experience of discontent in different ways, described it in detail, discussed its meaning for them, and spoke about their ways of coping with it, their successes and failures. It seems to me that the mere fact of discussing the problem out in the open, without attempting to prescribe detailed coping strategies, may be the beginning of a solution for people who reflect on their career as group care workers and how it affects their lives as people.

Although the book is also intended to reach researchers studying the social aspects of care and education and others concerned with youth care settings, its primary target audience consists of the group care workers themselves, those who are actually on the line in residential settings, as they reflect in private about their work, its challenges, and its difficulties and share with colleagues their experiences of discontent and how they deal with them. Thus, the book seeks to clarify the key questions that will, perhaps, help group care workers who reflect on their occupational and professional experiences to live into some of the answers.

WHY DISCONTENT?

Discontent is not an inevitable experience in the care of children and youth. Clearly, the encounter between the adult–the residential group care worker–and the youth can also lead to satisfying experiences. In fact, there is much evidence to show that residential care workers often enjoy their work and derive contentment from it. Nevertheless, several reasons led me to focus in this book mainly on aspects of discontent in direct care work.

My first reason for choosing to deal with discontent is personal experience. In my professional life I have been involved for almost 40 years, at least partially, in residential child and youth care. I have worked as a residential care worker, a teacher in a residential school, a supervisor of residential care workers (in an Israeli network of residential schools that specialize in the education of immigrant children and children from disadvantaged backgrounds), an instructor in the education and in-service training of residential care workers, a university lecturer teaching, among other things, the sociology of residential organizations, and a residential care researcher. During the early stages of my work in the field, I experienced discontent, the memory of which remains with me to this day.

My second reason for choosing this subject was my accumulated impression of discontent as I observed interactions between residential care workers and youth, and in talks with residential care workers over the years. It is my impression that all residential care workers have experienced discontent in varying degrees in the course of their careers.

Thus, I observed residential care workers in various age groups and from varied socioeconomic and cultural backgrounds in work situations that clearly did not give them satisfaction. During the interviews, some workers reported that the youth in their care cooperate with them much less than they expect; even worse, some of the workers complained that the youth ignored them; and worst of all, some youths and groups of youths, from time to time or throughout their stay in the setting, disrupt their work in ways that the residential care workers experience as rejection of their professionalism and humaneness.

My third reason for choosing to deal with discontent is the fact that the literature dealing with the study and interpretation of difficulties and conflicts in a related field, namely the school and its teaching staff, has for the past thirty years been dominant in the study of interactional sociology of the school and social psychology in education.[1]

The concept of "discontent" is not commonly used in the context of education or care; situations of difficulty in these domains are more commonly characterized as stress or burnout. These two terms have been described and defined in several ways.

The concept of stress usually relates to personal response. For example, the residential care worker is subject to stress or the victim of stress; stress affects the worker from within as a result of personality weaknesses, or from outside as a result of the circumstances of his or her work. The residential care worker is not the subject but the object of these effects. The concept of burnout often denotes the outcomes of stress: as a result of stress, the residential care worker experiences feelings of helplessness and failure whose effect is debilitating (Kyriacou, 1989).

Thus, these two concepts cast the teacher or residential care worker as a passive object and a victim–although perhaps at least partly to blame for his or her own plight–of organizational and occupational circumstances.

Rather than speaking of stress or burnout, therefore, I propose to discuss the phenomenon that I call discontent in care. I describe "discontent" as the residential care worker's continuous realization that unqualified, stable acceptance and cooperation on the part of his or her charges can never be gained. Such feelings of discontent may hamper or even paralyze residential care workers' functioning, and/or spur them to use means of coping whose purpose is to reduce the frustrating experience as much as possible.

My choice of the concept "discontent" was inspired by Freud's (1930) discussion of "Civilization and its Discontents," in which he presents civilization as a stimulating factor in human life that simultaneously creates distress. The experience of discontent hurts but does not necessarily paralyze; to a large extent, he observes, civilization is based on it. Likewise, it is common to discern a feeling of distress among teachers and residential care workers, but this sometimes acts simultaneously as a spur to their survival and their success in their work, stimulating them to persist in the same activity or to change their patterns of action. In other words, unlike stress and burnout, concepts that emphasize the residential care worker's passivity, "discontent" is neutral with regard to its causes and the anticipated response. Like man within civilization in Freud's essay, the residential care worker is in a state of discontent to which he or she may react either actively or passively.

"The Seasons of Our Discontent"

In pedagogic literature, states of discontent, by whatever names they are called, are sometimes presented as arising out of the educational workers' feeling that their influence on their charges is minimal. This situation may be described as resulting from the relatively meager material and symbolic (prestige, etc.) rewards that this work grants to the teacher or care worker. In some cases, it is presented as a result of the youths' limited ability to utilize the worker's contributions (to develop, to change, to form and develop an identity, to be rehabilitated), or of limitations inherent in the carers' caring ability and effectiveness.

The residential care workers whom we interviewed, however, emphasized in various ways the discontent arising out of their interactions with their charges. Discontent in caring will be discussed in the book mainly from this angle. Thus, our approach is an interactionist one. The world of the residential care worker is viewed as evolving largely through interaction, and the worker as "I being fulfilled in Thou" (Buber, 1958) through dialogues he or she conducts with significant "yous," the worker's charges. Investigation of the nature of these interactions is a major factor in studying the residential care worker's professional code.

THE INTERACTIONAL PROCESS

This approach is guided by the assumption that a person's world develops, exists, and changes primarily through his or her interactions with human partners. This is based on the argument that every social reality is largely a reflection of the tacit or overt agreements—usually transitory or changing—of people who meet together by virtue of a shared interest and therefore interact with each other.

As the process begins each of the participants enters a social situation (let us say, an evening meeting with the group) with his or her own interests and objectives and with at least some understanding of what is to take place. Usually, the individuals develop rational reasons as to how they can best further their own interests. In the course of interacting with the others, each individual negotiates over his or her interests and objectives vis-à-vis their interests and objectives and over his or her perception of the social reality developing between them. Thus, each individual attempts to persuade the others to accept his or her personal perceptions and on this basis to reach some kind of working consensus.

When a working consensus is achieved, all the parties will "behave" according to it until it is broken, when the interests and perceptions of one or more of those involved change, thus destroying the basis for the working consensus.

Such interactions are comprised of two major components: a *cognitive* aspect that is covert although surmisable or predictable by the partners, and an overt *behavioral* aspect. The cognitive aspect includes each individual's awareness of his or her interests and objectives, imputation of meaning to the situation, and his or her subjective understanding, evaluation, and choice of a course of action that will serve that person optimally. Sometimes the individual shares these actions with his or her "peers" through joint interpretive activity.

The behavioral element includes the individual's presentation of self (in such a way as to invite the others' supportive cooperation) and concrete negotiations, primarily through non-verbal gestures and discussion. Schematically the interaction can be depicted as in Figure 1. These aspects are mostly presented here not as a researcher's "impartial" view, but as the residential care workers themselves described them in reporting on their interactions with their most "significant others" or major "role complements" in the world of care: the young people in their care.

THE RESEARCH PROCESS

The present book describes phenomena that became manifest as patterns that recurred among many of the residential care workers we interviewed, phenomena that characterize residential care workers beyond their division into subgroups. With few exceptions, it does not discuss groups differentiated on such variables as gender, length of tenure, specific role in direct care, or type or level of residential school. The residential care workers' world that emerges from these discussions appears to cut across the boundaries of such classifications and subdivisions.

FIGURE 1. Structure of Interaction

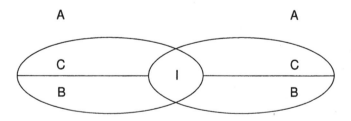

A = acting (action) = cognitively-based behavior
C = cognizing
B = behaving
I = interacting

The residential care worker's "role partners"–residential care work colleagues, advisors, and the youth in his or her care–are described where this seems to be necessary. In very rare cases it was decided to present the interviewer's direct impressions as well.

Thus, our main data source is a study consisting of 37 interviews with residential care workers. The interviews began with a general presentation and clarification of their purpose: to obtain descriptions and evaluations of the interviewee's interactions with his or her charges.

However, these in-depth interviews were conducted without pre-arranged specification as to what questions to ask the workers and at what stages of the interview; although we possessed, particularly in the more advanced stages, a list of subjects that interested us, in most cases we avoided asking specific and direct questions. The only subject introduced by us in every case when the interviewee did not bring it up was the possibility of "improper behavior" of the youth towards the worker or his or her colleagues.

Every interview explains something from another interview and, in turn, is explained to some degree by another interview. Each interprets and is interpreted in the framework of the unifying text. Thus, the importance of these combinations does not lie in their expanding the store of knowledge but in reading the data anew and increasing their ability to explain.

The interviews focused on distinct aspects of the interactions between residential care workers and their role partners. However, they do not document planned and supervised interactions in "laboratory conditions" nor specific, well-defined variables. Their point of departure was ethnographic and holistic, often leading the interviews into rich "digressions" that illuminated aspects that emerged or had emerged in other interviews.

Thus, the materials presented here are not reports of direct observation of interactions between residential care workers and youth. Not only was the cognitive aspect–the intentions and evaluations–of the residential care worker and his charges hidden but, in the nature of studies based on interviews, the behavioral aspect of the interaction was not overt, either. Working on the basis of unstructured interviews means that the conclusions depend to a large extent on retrospective or "post factum" reports, reports made after the interactions described had concluded.

The guiding concept was that the basis for obtaining the knowledge sought is knowledge of the actors, in our case, residential care workers, and their role partners. In principle, it is assumed here that the information offered by the actors and its accompanying explanation is no less valid than the interviewer's knowledge. Furthermore, as Eisikovits (1991) and Weiner (1991) have demonstrated, in principle the interviewed residential care workers could have functioned as their own reflective ethnographers and interpreters of the action in which they participated.

However, I preferred materials emerging in open interviews over data arising out of self-reflective reports of actors or obtained by processing the responses to a structured questionnaire. This approach is inherent in the nature of the central question, the question of discontent in care. Reliance on the residential care workers' self-reports of their situation in interactions with their charges is based on the assumption that residential care workers are prepared to report openly on the extent of their discontent and their problems at work. But many residential care workers tend to avoid admitting the existence of these phenomena or to minimize their extent because of the fear of becoming stigmatized.

In open interviews, on the other hand, we could let the residential care workers speak about their problems at their own pace and scope, and thus encourage them to share their problems with us. It was not our impression that our interviewees always met, or could meet, the condition set by Searle (1984): "The explanation of an action must have the same content as was in the person's head when he performed the action or when he reasoned toward his intention to perform the action" (p. 67). The open interview situation actually allowed the workers to avoid discussing embarrassing personal experiences by displacing them, consciously or otherwise, to a discussion of the experiences of residential care workers in general or of specific colleagues.

Our research taught us once again what we had learned before from such observers as Geerts (1975) and Schutz (1970): We never describe "objective" social realities; rather, we perform a subjective function—we interpret. Our interviewees interpreted their reality and that of their colleagues. We interpret their interpretations. In turn, readers will hopefully interpret our interpretations of the interviewees' interpretations.

On the whole, however, their reports did not seem to be interest-guided distortions or loaded with purely ideological justifications, although it was certainly not always possible to regard the reports as necessarily valid in themselves. Sometimes we got the impression that the information we were given was more important as a source of knowledge about the respondent than about the event being described. In such cases, it seemed more appropriate to prefer an alternative version offered by the researcher (and, of course, identified as such).

OVERVIEW

Chapter 1 opens with a description of the residential care worker and the social organization in which he or she functions ("The Setting and the

Role"). The model is the Israeli one, which undoubtedly differs in many ways from models of workers and settings in other countries and cultures. But again, both the worker and the setting have some major characteristics that I have reason to believe cross cultural boundaries. I have tried to the best of my ability to present aspects beyond the specific Israeli culture at the center of the discussion. Nevertheless, I see no need to avoid, nor can I avoid, presenting some unique and idiosyncratic characteristics of the Israeli worker and setting when this seems to be called for.

The next four chapters are devoted to detailed descriptions by residential care workers of situations they perceive as situations of discontent. Chapter 2 deals with their perceptions of the care situation and particularly of the power of the youth, which they feel is often directed against them ("Situations"). The following chapter discusses the workers' perception of the identity of the youth who hurt them or in different ways cause them (or their colleagues) discontent ("Who Hurts?"). Chapter 4 deals with their perception of the identity of those of their colleagues who are particularly vulnerable to being hurt by their charges ("Who Is Hurt?"). Chapter 5 asks what kinds of actions or inactions on the part of the youth cause the most discontent among workers ("What Hurts?").

Following these discussions of the residential care workers' perceptions of situations of discontent, Chapter 6 deals with the question of what strategies they use to control their charges' behavior so as to enable them, the workers, to cope with their situation and survive at work ("The Residential Setting as a Negotiated Order"). I wish to stress that the description is not of effective, prescribable strategies, but of those that are actually employed, irrespective of the issue of their actual effectiveness.

Chapter 7, which concludes the volume, summarizes the nature of the experience of discontent and reflects on residential care workers' chances of coping effectively with the situations of discontent in which they find themselves ("Care, Contentment, and Commitment").

NOTES

1. The literature on difficulties and conflicts in teaching is extensive and varied. This work was directly inspired and influenced by descriptions in books and papers that follow interactionist and conflict traditions (Ball, 1987; Blase, 1991; Cole & Walker, 1989; Denscombe, 1985; Hargreaves, Hester, & Mellor, 1975; Malen,1994; Tyler, 1988; Woods, 1990; Woods & Pollard, 1988).

About two years before the completion of the present book, I published a book in Hebrew, *Teaching and its Discontents* (Arieli, 1995). To some extent, that research was conducted on teachers and residential care workers together. More precisely, the ethnographic work on residential care workers began in 1985, five years before I started collecting ethnographic data on secondary school teachers. However, the analysis of the teacher data, as well as the writing and publication of that book, preceded the analysis and write-up of the residential care worker data.

Teaching and its Discontents was largely an inductive work; I derived the structure of the book primarily from my field notes. The structuring of The *Occupational Experience of Residential Child and Youth Care Workers: Caring and Its Discontents* was modelled in part on the same framework, since both studies concern the subject of discontent among workers in educational organizations and both deal with interaction between educators and those being educated. While reading the ethnographic materials for the present book, I found that the content of the two studies resembled each other much more than I had assumed; both are studies of people-processing organizations that confront adults with adolescents (and the reverse). I decided, therefore, that despite the ethnographic character of the residential care study, it would be well served by using parts of the structure of my previous book on teachers.

Chapter 1

The Setting and the Role

Before discussing the daily experiences of residential care workers in their interactions with their charges, let us take a look at the arena and the actors. The discussion of the setting and the people will deal with "generalized" organizations and people, namely, with those organizational and human characteristics that cross the boundaries of a specific culture.

Although it is doubtful whether such "general" persons and organizations actually exist, a scrutiny of the relevant literature demonstrates that many of the major characteristics of organizations and people recur in similar patterns in many cultures.[2] This, in my view, justifies generalized descriptions of the organization and its staff. Since the ethnographic data to be presented are derived from the reality of role bearers and settings in one specific culture, the Israeli culture, however, it seems appropriate to include a short explanation of these organizations and role bearers in Israel as well.

I shall thus first discuss the nature of residential care settings in general, followed by some remarks on residential care settings in Israel. Thirdly, I shall present a description of the universal elements in the roles of residential care workers as reflected in many different cultures.[3] I will conclude with a description of the specific nature of the roles of residential care workers in Israel (the madrich and the em-bayit).

RESIDENTIAL CARE SETTINGS

Residential care settings are places where young people spend all or most of their time, often for several years of their lives, in varying degrees of organized separation both from their original community and from the social environment around these settings. The long, continuous stay in one

[Haworth co-indexing entry note]: "The Setting and The Role." Arieli, Mordecai. Co-published simultaneously in *Child & Youth Services* (The Haworth Press, Inc.) Vol. 18, No. 2, 1997, pp. 11-22; and: *The Occupational Experience of Residential Child and Youth Care Workers: Caring and Its Discontents* (Mordecai Arieli) The Haworth Press, Inc., 1997, pp. 11-22. Single or multiple copies of this article are available for a fee from The Haworth Document Delivery Service [1-800-342-9678, 9:00 a.m. - 5:00 p.m. (EST). E-mail address: getinfo@haworth.com].

11

place and the isolation from society are regarded as assets that help the residential setting to achieve whatever educational and socialization aims are determined by its founders and management.

The assumption is that the setting exerts pressure on its residents to adapt and internalize pre-selected, structured modes of behavior and sets of norms through constant exposure to these influences and because of the advantageous position the residential setting has relative to the influences of the social structures outside its walls. This pressure on the youth–operated as a strategy for change and achieved by means of controlled isolation and exposure–justifies the description of the residential care setting as a powerful environment (Arieli, Kashti, & Shlasky, 1983).

Care and education in residential settings is made available for various age groups (young children, adolescents, the old) and for people with other special social identities, often deviant (handicapped, sick, or delinquent, as opposed to "regular" adolescents, for example). The present study relates only to residential settings for young people and their staffs. Settings of this kind form a broad category and are very varied, reflecting differing sets of structural and management variables. Some of the significant factors distinguishing among various types of residential settings for children and youth follow.

1. Size

The size of such settings ranges from family-type settings for perhaps eight children to large programs with well over 200 residents. Size clearly affects the number of staff members and the structure and definition of their roles.

2. Type of Service Provided

Is the setting primarily educational? Is it designed mainly for youngsters from social elites, the mainstream, or less privileged classes? Does it offer the kind of formal education customarily provided by the state to youth who can be described as regular, or is it a setting whose main purpose is to give shelter, care, and treatment, to youth with problematic or "deviant" social identities? What is the proportion of workers of various kinds in the residential setting, and how does this affect the character of the staff culture?

3. Scope of Services Provided

Does the setting provide all the services needed by the youth? What aspects of life are covered by the services provided? To what outside services–if any–does it refer its residents? Does the setting have a school, or are the residents sent to schools in the neighboring community? To what extent does the residential setting constitute a total life situation?

4. Links with Neighboring Communities

Often, youth in residential settings attend school in the surrounding community. Alternatively, some residential settings include a school that may also enroll students from the neighboring community, perhaps even serving as a comprehensive school for the entire region. In other cases it serves only the residents of the setting. Who, then, are the clients of the residential setting's staff–the residential children alone, or perhaps also children and youth from the neighboring community as well (Shapira, 1987)?

5. Unifying Culture

To what extent do the staff members share a common culture: values, outlook (religious, ideological), educational or care orientation, and social or professional viewpoint? If there is a unifying culture, the staff members act as agents of that culture with a high level of mutual commitment, whereas in the absence of a unifying culture they may perceive themselves as people hired to do a job, not particularly involved in the basic values represented, usually, by the head.

6. Autonomy of the Residential Setting as an Administrative and Economic Entity

Some residential settings belong to national or other public networks that are responsible for their budgets and in some cases actually manage the setting. Other residential settings, although formally belonging to national or regional networks, have to find their own funding and administer their budgets themselves. An important question is to what extent the staff run the setting. Also, how much time can the staff, and particularly the head, spare from bargaining for resources for the organization to administer the educational and care work (Meyer, Scott, & Deal, 1983)?

7. Living Together

The youth in a residential setting are there day and night. Depending on the setting, however, sometimes all the staff members, sometimes most of them, and sometimes just a few choose (and are allowed) to bring their families and make their own homes in the setting or nearby, on the grounds. Thus, the youth and staff members often constitute one geographical community. Both members of a couple may work in the setting in various roles. Thus, the lives of resident staff members are often largely exposed to colleagues and to the youth even outside working hours.

In these circumstances, relations with the youth may cross the dividing lines between primary and secondary relationships, between professional or work relationships and friendship (Davies-Jones, 1985). In the family-style home, the children sit around the breakfast table with the workers and their children, or they spend the evening watching TV together in the family living room. In a large residential setting, the head and his or her spouse, whether they like it or not, may also serve as models of family relations for the staff members and their charges.

How does one live in this situation of (at least potential) mutual exposure? Should one draw a line between formal, bureaucratic, work relations and friendship? Is it all right for the head to convene a staff meeting at his or her home? Is it appropriate, particularly in view of the distance from the neighboring community, for a staff member to "pop in" to a neighbor who may be his or her supervisee for a glass of beer in the evening or to ask a child to run an errand? In the circumstances of the residential setting, to what extent can one be both an equal and a superior?

RESIDENTIAL SETTINGS: THE ISRAELI WAY

Many children and youth in Israel are placed in residential programs. During the 1994-1995 school year, 39,700 young people were served in the 234 residential educational and child and youth care facilities supervised by the Ministry of Education that were operating in Israel. In the past decade approximately 40,000 youth aged 13-18 were in such settings each year, comprising about 11% of the entire pupil population in that age range (Central Bureau of Statistics, 1996). During the past quarter century there were years when almost 20% of the 13-18 age group were in residential settings.

The popularity of residential settings in Israel has deep historical and social roots. For generations, the most prestigious program of Jewish education in the Diaspora was the yeshiva (Talmudic or post-Biblical Jewish institution of higher learning). For most students, attending a yeshiva entailed leaving home, since many Jewish communities were too small to run their own yeshivas.

The yeshiva fulfilled two purposes in traditional Jewish society. It served both as an elite educational institution and as a route of social mobility for members of lower social classes. This was possible because gifted, motivated pupils were generally admitted regardless of their social backgrounds. Although most yeshiva institutions did not provide residential facilities, life away from home boarding with local families, like life in formal residential settings, was legitimized by Jewish communities.

In pre-state Israel (before 1948), residential agricultural schools as well as kibbutzim often operated as residential centers for youth from central and eastern Europe who came to the country singly or in groups aiming to revolutionize traditional patterns of Jewish life. For the indigenous children, the role of these schools was to support and accelerate socialization toward membership in the group to which they belonged by birth. For immigrant youth, the role of these settings was more in the nature of resocialization, an attempt to bring about changes in their original social ization (Kashti, 1988)

CARING WHILE SCHOOLING: THE CAREGIVERS' APPROACH

In the early 1970s it was established that a great number of children of new immigrants were not doing well at school. They were often labelled as educationally disadvantaged. It was suggested that many so-called disadvantaged youth show symptoms of maladjustment as well: various deviancies and problems of mental health. It was also believed that the disadvantaged would benefit from residential programs.

The underlying assumption was that exposing disadvantaged children and youth and those requiring extra-familial care to the daily influence of a setting that operates as a cultural agent of society may, over a period of years, help to advance their academic achievement and to rehabilitate them socially and psychologically at the same time.

The pioneering idea of residential schooling was gradually replaced by the two ideas of normalization and mainstreaming. Thus, Israeli policy makers began to view residential schooling as a means of bringing young members of marginal groups toward the social center as well as a way of caring for youngsters with various social and psychological problems.

Approximately 80-90% of the 40,000 young people who are placed in Israeli residential settings today are in organizations known as youth villages and boarding schools. These are characterized mainly by the following features.

First, all aspects of the residents' lives take place in one framework. They spend their leisure time, sleep, and study on the same campus; there is no distinction between school and home.

Second, the school is conducted as a regular day school. In fact, it often serves as a day school for local youth who are not boarders in the residential setting.

Third, these are large settings, accommodating 100 to 600 youth in residence.

Fourth, the official orientation guiding the settings is that of schooling—the staff's main role is to teach, while the children's main purpose is to study. The idea of care is subordinate to that of education.

There is growing awareness that the youth are often sent to settings because of social or psychological distress, but the challenges facing the staff and the youth are normative ones: success in studies and mainstreaming.

The other 10-20% of youth in residential settings are in settings defined as care, treatment, or rehabilitation organizations. These are small settings, usually with no more than 100 residents, who often attend schools outside the campus.

To sum up, one may say that the dominant approach in the residential network is: "We care while we school." The residents quietly receive care while openly taking part in what they and the adults in charge of them identify as education. There is fairly broad agreement in educational and professional circles in Israel concerning the advantages of the approach that puts education before care when dealing with children and youth who are diagnosed as needing to be taken away from their homes, whether temporarily or permanently.[4]

RESIDENTIAL CARE WORKERS:
"LOCALS" AND "COSMOPOLITANS"

The staffs of Israeli residential settings usually include semi-professional residential care workers as well as professional educational counselors, teachers, social workers, and psychologists. This is a multi-disciplinary staff with a variety of roles that differ in many aspects. Two related aspects merit brief discussion: the clarity of the roles and their boundaries, and the source of staff members' professional authority.

The role of the residential care worker is often diffuse and ambiguous: what is included in the role and what is not? Each residential care worker has to deal with support and discipline, encouraging the individual and guiding the group, and supervising and preparing events (Carlebach, 1982; Waaldijk, 1994). The residential care worker often has to help with homework and is responsible for order and cleanliness, taking care of the youth's clothes and so forth.

Similarly, the extent of the residential care workers' authority–what they are allowed to do and what they are forbidden to do with regard to their charges–is somewhat vague. They are generally overworked; they are also required to possess a great deal of information about the youngsters' backgrounds, what the teachers and other educators expect of their students, and the like.

The tasks of the teacher, psychologist, social worker, and educational counselor, on the other hand, are relatively clear and well defined. The teacher teaches in the classroom; the others deal with diagnosis and therapy or guidance. True, these professionals are expected (and expect themselves) to function in a more generalized manner–not just to teach a subject but to "educate"; not to be a psychological "technician" but a holistic therapist. Nevertheless, their role definitions are not so vague, and less is expected of them.

The tasks of the semi-professional residential care workers are largely determined inside the residential setting where they work, mainly by their direct superiors. A comparison of the role content and authority of the group care worker in different settings within the country, even in the same region, often yields substantial differences. Furthermore, in a large residential setting there are often considerable differences between the head's definition of the residential care worker's role and authority and the group care coordinator's perception of the same role. In contrast, the roles of the psychologist, teacher, social worker, and educational counselor are largely defined outside the residential setting, in universities and professional associations, and shaped by factors outside the settings in which they work.

Following Gouldner (1970), we can refer to those whose role is defined mainly in the organization in which they work (here, the residential care workers) as "locals," and those whose role is defined primarily by factors independent of the employing organization as "cosmopolitans." The "locals" are competent to work mainly in their "local" organization, largely on the basis of experience acquired there. The "cosmopolitans," at least on the face of it, can practice their profession anywhere. The former feel that they are expected to do "everything" for meager symbolic and material rewards; the latter try to restrict themselves as far as possible to their area of expertise and to be paid as "specialists."

In residential settings, the "locals" often live in the setting, while the "cosmopolitans" are not generally to be found among its residents or on the grounds after their working hours. The former work long hours (with some exaggeration, "day and night") and often perceive themselves as more involved in their charges' lives than the latter.

The various role bearers in the residential setting, both "locals" and "cosmopolitans," share in professional cultures either inside or outside the residential setting. These cultures form values pertaining to issues concerning workers' participation in decision-making processes in the organization. Observation in several Israeli residential settings and interviews with staff members confirm my impression that the "locals" tend to differ from the "cosmopolitans" in terms of their values and expectations in this regard.

Some of the "locals" expect to be included in the decision making process, at least as advice-givers, though there are some who prefer to limit their involvement to those areas in which they work directly. The latter tend to expect a more authoritarian style of management than do their more "involved" colleagues and the "cosmopolitans." The "cosmopolitans" usually insist on participating in decision making, not only as advisors but also as rightful partners in a democratic process, or as professionals whose expertise qualifies them to share in decisions concerning their field.

The dilemma often faced by the head of the residential setting is whether and in what circumstances to meet the staff's expectations concerning his or her style of management. It might seem that the "locals'" lack of or more limited professional training justifies their exclusion from decision making processes, while the "cosmopolitans'" professionalism justifies their inclusion in these processes (Goldman & Manburg, 1985). On the other hand, failure to include the "locals" in the process is apt to lead to alienation among those who wish to be involved and to cause those who are not so inclined to adopt a stance of indifference. And regular inclusion of the "cosmopolitans" in the decision making process might lead to the forming of coalitions against the head and weaken his or her status.

Reddin (1970), in the framework of his tri-dimensional managerial theory, suggests that there is no ideal managerial style but that the manager has to diagnose the demands of the situation and adapt his or her managerial style accordingly. A staff of workers whose roles require considerable skill, professionalism, and creativity tends to demand autonomy in choosing work methods, if only because the staff's knowledge—each one in his or her field—often exceeds that of the head. This kind of staff tends to reject close control. A staff of workers with limited skill whose work is routine and repetitive and whose director's knowledge exceeds that of the members usually expects a great deal of guidance and even control.

But what is the appropriate managerial style for the head in a complex organizational situation where some of the staff belong to the first category and some to the second? Can the head of the residential setting adopt a dual managerial style, encouraging autonomy among some of the staff and keeping tight control over the others, particularly when the "locals" occupy an essential role in the operation that requires a great deal of skill and initiative?[5]

THE MADRICH AND THE EM-BAYIT

In Israel, a male residential care worker called a *madrich* (a word that means leader or guide) typically works side by side with a female worker called an *em-bayit* (housemother). This division of the work between the two genders apparently has its source in the wish of the founders of residential schools in the 1930s and '40s to have parent-like figures fulfilling the traditional roles of parents for uprooted children and war refugees. In the past decade, a discernible effort has been made to unify these two roles. One expression of this is evident in in-service and other training courses for people in both roles, where all are, if only for the duration of the courses, called "residential educational workers." In recent years, the role of madrich is sometimes given to a woman (madricha).

The Madrich

The madrich is expected to be at the disposal of his charges during all the daytime hours that are not devoted to formal activity (e.g., schooling), that is to say, at mealtimes and the times set for looking after their things, cleaning their dormitories, doing homework, social activities, and leisure time. The nature of the youths' activities during the time they are supervised by the madrich indicates the wide variety of his or her role components, requiring both a developmental and a custodial orientation toward the young people, relating simultaneously to the individual and the group.

Until the mid-1970s, the madrich was mainly expected to help individual youth cope with the many and often conflicting expectations directed at them in the residential setting, the differential and complex nature of which made it difficult for many of the young people to meet all of their needs. It was the task of the madrich to harmonize the residents with the setting and to help maintain an equilibrium between them.

According to Goffman (1961), one of the characteristics of the total institution that undermines the inmates' identity is their dependence on a large, complex and clumsy apparatus to satisfy their smallest needs. Therefore, an educational organization with total characteristics needs a figure who can help the residents to maintain the integration of their personalities. Until recently, the general expectation in the Israeli residential setting was that this would be done by the madrich.

Although in recent years this function has been gradually passing from the madrich to the professional worker, the madrich is still expected to view the youths as complete personalities and to relate to them in a diffuse and particularistic manner. In this sense the madrich's role resembles that of a father. Alongside this parental function, however, the madrich is expected to perform individual developmental functions, group developmental functions, individual custodial functions, and group custodial functions (Shlasky, 1985). Official documents prescribing the role of the madrich emphasize a preference for the developmental rather than the custodial aspect, both in the number of role components and in the force of the demands they make upon the madrich.

The emphasis in the role of the madrich in Israeli residential settings has actually changed twice. During the 1930s and '40s, the social component was considered the major one; the madrich was perceived as the central factor in recruiting the youth to the ideology of a pioneering settlement. From the 1950s on, when the political "ideological" education systems were replaced by the State education system with its strong achievement orientation alongside the increasing penetration of approaches stressing the child's well-being, the individual component of the madrich's role was increasingly emphasized above the social one. This emphasis was reflected in the large amount of time devoted by the madrich to helping with homework and to individual supportive talks.

Since the mid-1970s, another change has appeared in the madrich's role. Helping with homework is gradually being taken out of the hands of the madrichim, either because they are not sufficiently equipped with knowledge of the subject matter taught in the secondary school or because they are not trained in the didactic techniques required for helping students with learning problems. Also, in many residential settings, there has been a growth of groups, including study groups, run by specialists who are not regular members of the staff.

As a result, the individual youth joins in many such activities, thus reducing the extent of his direct contacts with the madrichim. This process intensifies with the entrance of professional workers: clinical school psychologists, educational counselors, and social workers, who are expected to provide a large amount of the support that previously came from the madrich. This makes the madrich largely a supervisor of the youths' participation in the various activities.

The Em-Bayit

The em-bayit (housemother) complements the madrich in charge of one of the educational groups in the residential setting. Her role prescriptions include caring for the youths' personal cleanliness, for the cleanliness and tidiness of their rooms, their health and clothing, their eating habits and nourishment, and also their general feelings of well-being.

Together with the madrich, the housemother is expected to see that the group members get up in the morning. She then supervises them in making their beds, cleaning their rooms, and going to the dining room for breakfast. During these early morning hours, her hands are full urging on those who do not want to get up and looking after sick youngsters or sending them to the clinic.

Until mid-day the em-bayit supervises youths who are on rota duty cleaning the dormitories (clubroom, corridors, washrooms), attends to the group's laundry, their clothing repairs, and the care of the store-room. She eats lunch with her charges and in some residential settings supervises or helps with the serving of meals.

In some residential settings the housemother and the madrich together hold a weekly group meeting to discuss the group's social and organizational problems. In many settings the em-bayit replaces the madrich one evening a week, devising some kind of leisure activity with the youths for that evening.

The em-bayit's role prescriptions and work schedule show that she is expected to respond to two kinds of needs of the residents: adaptive needs and tension-release needs. The desire to meet these two types of needs through one role-bearer is drawn from the model of the family. The em-bayit is perceived as the mother of the group.

The need to respond to these two groups of needs has led to the formation of two basic concepts of the em-bayit's role vis-à-vis the youths: the service-custodial approach, expressed in role components such as keeping order, cleanliness, and the timetable; and the formative-development approach, expressed in components such as caring for the youths' well-being and comfort and having supportive talks with individuals. These two approaches emphasize the diffuse, obscure and often conflicting aspects of the em-bayit's role.

It sometimes happens that the housemother gets involved in conflicts resulting from the contradiction between her personal perception of her role and the way it is perceived by her superiors. While she perceives her role primarily as a formative-developmental one, she feels that her superiors expect her to devote herself primarily to the service-custodial aspects. Sometimes the formal role prescriptions support the formative role concept of the housemother, but the custodial norms which actually prevail in the residential setting contradict this.

The conflict between the formative and custodial aspects of the house-mother's role appears to be particularly pressing because the custodial aspects are overt and convenient for definition, expectation, and reward, while the formative role components exist mainly as an approach and not as clear definitions of performance.

While the average duration of employment of a madrich is three to four years and they are mostly young men in their twenties, em-bayits remain in their jobs for an average of about fifteen years and their ages range widely. The fact that an em-bayit is often many years older than the madrich with whom she works—as well as much older than the youths—is regarded by many of the older em-bayits as a problem (Shalom, 1980; Arieli, Kashti, & Shlasky, 1983; Shlasky, 1985; Eisikovits, Z., 1986).

NOTES

2. Multicultural descriptions have recently been offered, for example, by Bullock, Little, and Millham (1993), Colton and Hellinckx (1993), and Gottesmann (1991b, 1994). Sociological analyses of the international scene have been offered by Kashti (1988, 1991). Descriptions of settings and systems in particular countries which are relevant to the present discussion have been offered by Adler and Shapira (1981), Arieli, Kashti, and Shlasky (1983), Feuerstein (1987), and Wozner (1991) on the Israeli scene; Beker (1981) and VanderVen (1991) on the US scene; Anglin (1991) on the Canadian scene; Bullock (1993), Kahan (1994), Lane (1994), and Little (1995) on the British scene; and Frommann, Haag, and Trede (1991) and Colla-Müller (1993) on the German scene.

3. The English term for this role: residential care worker or residential child care worker, is prevalent in the UK (alongside other names such as residential worker and residential social worker). In the USA the terms generally used are residential counsellor, child–and/or youth–care worker, and cottage parent. In countries outside the English speaking world similar terms are used. Further details on the names of the bearers of the role appear in the FICE International Bulletin (1990).

4. For a comparison of key themes in Israeli residential programs with those in such programs in the United States, see Beker and Magnuson (1996).

5. On the professionalization of child care staff see also Powell (1990), Kelly (1990), and Gottesmann (1991a).

Chapter 2

The Situations

From the point of view of the actors (the residential care workers, the youth in care, and all the others), residential settings exist as an ongoing series of situations. Each actor experiences, understands, or defines the situations that arise subjectively, although sometimes a group of actors who share a common status form a common perspective that leads to the formulation of an intersubjective definition of the situation.

Thus, the definition of the situation is the subjective meaning ascribed by an individual or group of individuals to events happening in the social reality of which they are a part. This approach is guided by W.I. Thomas's (1972) well-known observation that if people define situations as real, then they are real in their consequences.[6]

In his[7] daily work the residential care worker shares in many situations that vary in their structure and content as well as in the number of other participants and other factors. Most of the situations that he takes part in, or finds himself in, are shared with his charges. In the context of these situations he interacts with them—it may be a single youth, a random group of youth, or the whole formal group under his care. In most of these interactions he is the only adult; sometimes he works with another adult, other residential care workers, or professionals in educational or behavioral work.

Most of the situations he shares with his charges are informal ones, but in many residential settings—in most of those in Israel, for example—he allots one or two evenings a week to scheduled group discussions. These are activities of a somewhat formal nature devoted to group matters or to discussing news and current topics, and all the group members are usually required to attend.

[Haworth co-indexing entry note]: "The Situations." Arieli, Mordecai. Co-published simultaneously in *Child & Youth Services* (The Haworth Press, Inc.) Vol. 18, No. 2, 1997, pp. 23-31; and: *The Occupational Experience of Residential Child and Youth Care Workers: Caring and Its Discontents* (Mordecai Arieli) The Haworth Press, Inc., 1997, pp. 23-31. Single or multiple copies of this article are available for a fee from The Haworth Document Delivery Service [1-800-342-9678, 9:00 a.m. - 5:00 p.m. (EST). E-mail address: getinfo@haworth.com].

23

The residential care worker possesses previous generalized knowledge of his group and specific knowledge with regard to some of its members. This includes his perceptions and images of their power, their state of mind, and their ability, as individuals and as a collective, to constrain and control his behavior. And similarly, they have previous knowledge and understanding concerning their friends and peers, their workers, and the powers that these parties can exert on them. Every new encounter brings new impressions of what is anticipated in the situation that is about to unfold. These impressions are dynamic and changeable; many things can happen in an encounter before it ends.

PUBLIC AND PRIVATE DEFINITIONS OF THE SITUATION

The definition of the situation by an individual acting in a social context–for our purposes, the residential care worker–has two aspects: public and private/intimate. The public definition of the situation is expressed directly and indirectly, verbally and non-verbally, in front of the partners to the interaction–the youth in care, etc. It is presented with the intention of persuading or coercing, in the hope that it will be adopted as others' definition of the situation, too, thus ensuring their cooperation.

> *Asher:*[8] I told them straight in the face, "Five girls were late for kitchen duty again. O.K., I can easily fix it for you to spend the weekend here [when most would normally have passes]. There are plenty of things here that need cleaning, and people who get out of doing their chores can make up for it over the weekend ... " Then I said, "Donna, what are you smiling about? We'll see how you smile on Saturday when everyone else but you and a few other jokers have gone home. You too, Nancy. We don't force anyone to behave themselves here, but chores have to be done. It's not a right, it's a must. Is that clear?" It was very clear to them.
>
> Madrichim [plural of madrich] sometimes have to pressure them. Sometimes you have to spell things out loud and clear ... I know people say it is not pedagogically correct and the boss doesn't always like it, but in these things you usually have no trouble getting the people at the top to back you up.

Usually a few of the youths grumble, but in these circumstances, especially since the support of management is apparently guaranteed, the residential care worker's definition of the situation is accepted or, perhaps, successfully enforced.

Private or intimate definitions of the situation include, among other things, the residential care worker's evaluation of such matters as his charges' opinion of his ability to arouse their interest, their tendency to cooperate with him (for example, to take part in group discussions), their ability to oppose his plans, and his power to persuade them, to constrain their responses, or to coerce them to cooperate. Such assessments will strongly affect his choice of public behaviors as events unfold and the course of action he chooses to achieve the cooperation of the youth. They will influence the way he presents himself to them, and his way of responding to and developing the situation, and hence, the "outcomes."

These intimate definitions of the situation take place hidden from sight, as it were, between the individual and himself alone. But the partners to the interaction and external observers may be aware of them or discover them partly or fully as they decode the verbal and body language of the actor (the individual observed in action) during an incident and as they interpret it, that is, impute meanings to it. After the event, the actor and the observer may discuss the intimate definition of the situation.

Benny: Shuki went out to town again without permission. He disappeared for about ten hours. According to the rules, I should have reported it at once to the chief madrich, but that would have stirred up a lot of trouble. There's no messing around when a kid skips out. Once a girl who went missing for five hours was thrown out of the setting altogether. Shuki's in trouble with the chief madrich already, and with a lot of other people, too. I didn't want to get him into any more trouble, even though I risked my own skin in the process. I was very worried about his disappearance. He's very adventurous and always getting into scrapes. You never know where he is and what he might be doing.

It was a relief when he came back, but I still had a problem. The whole group knew he had taken off–Shuki himself made sure of that! Now they were waiting to see what I would do.

That evening we had the regular group meeting. Shuki sat there among his groupies, beaming in triumph. You could hear a lot of giggling and half-hidden mocking of me. I knew they were waiting to see how I would react. I could have ignored it, but looking at their faces I knew that if I didn't come down hard on Shuki I would lose an important battle. Suddenly I found strength I didn't know I had. I started screaming at him, and it worked. The bunch of groupies shut up, somewhat shocked. Shuki–I would never have believed this–lowered his eyes.

I had read the map right. I can't say that since then Shuki has become a kitten, but he hasn't been a tiger, either.

Batia: I have noticed that I often stop in the middle of talking to the youngsters and wonder what they think of me. Do they want to be like me, or am I something that's not really worth imitating? How much do they identify with what I represent? How consistent and strong am I and how far can I stand up to the pressures and threats and still keep going? The constant testing is like being under a magnifying glass–every movement, every look, every word, is scrutinized. I try to make sure they get the right impression of me. Often I feel they think of me as "the establishment," one of those . . . something to keep away from, to distrust.

DISRUPTIONS AND HURTS

The residential care workers used various expressions to describe behaviors that they identified as making them or their colleagues feel uncomfortable. A term commonly used was "disruption," denoting action that disrupts the course of a meeting, makes the worker's work harder, but does not hurt him. Another common term was "hurt." This is action that residential care workers identified as emotionally painful, often describing it as resulting from deliberate action.

"Disruption" and "hurt" are not "objective" situations or characteristics but the subjective definitions of someone who experiences them in a given situation, in this case the residential care worker.[9] Thus, "disruption" or disturbance and "hurt" served the interviewees mainly to denote experience whose meaning is subjective.

Kedem: It disturbs me that this overgrown lad is not prepared to wash . . . He's never outright cheeky, he doesn't give cocky answers. He just doesn't get washed . . . And when I dare to tell him again he smiles at me condescendingly to calm me down. Why does it bother me that he doesn't wash? Really, you might think it's my business! Once he said to me, "My girlfriend doesn't think I stink. She just thinks I'm not clean. If it doesn't bother her, why should it bother you?"

In some sense he's right. But it disturbs me very much. You ask if it disturbs other residential care workers. Look, according to the rules the kids have to wash, but maybe not all the residential care workers consider it a personal disturbance when a boy doesn't do it.

Dan: I think the girl didn't mean to hurt Shula (the em-bayit) at all, but Shula is very vulnerable; everything hurts her. That's her personality; it's not that there was any real intention to hurt.

However, other interviewees spoke of experiences that were clearly painful. These behaviors were usually described as "lack of respect" or even "humiliation."

> *Daniella*: I felt as if they couldn't care less what I said. "You told us, so what? We'll smoke if we want to. What will you do to us?"

> *Claire*: I asked a child to help me move some benches. This is a boy I've known for 5 years, since he was six, and I'm quite fond of him. He said, "Get lost, old woman!" I was horrified, but I didn't give up. Then he said, "Go do it yourself. That's what you're paid for, isn't it"? I don't know if he did it deliberately to hurt me or whether it was just an outburst in a moment of anger and frustration, but in any case I felt very humiliated. Why should he talk like that to someone who's devoted to him?

> *Ephraim*: When I got angry they parroted my words, while the rest of the group served as their audience, laughing at me. What I felt then can be described as utter humiliation: 10- and 11-year-old children making me look like a fool.

The expressions that recurred most often in the interviews with the residential care workers were "disruption" and "hurt." These words indicate a variety of behaviors that arouse feelings of discontent among many of the workers but not all of them. In their public definitions of situations of encounters with their charges, and also in seeking to "convince" the interviewer of their version of the meaning of what had happened in those encounters, the residential care workers referred to the identity, characteristics, and motives of the young people underlying their emotionally painful "disrupting" and, particularly, "hurting" behavior.

The emphasis, however, was often on the experience of the person who was hurt and the feeling of hurt and its meanings. Interviewees repeated some of their own intimate definitions of situations they had encountered during difficult moments in the clubroom, or attributed meaning to intimate definitions of situations as they were defined by fellow residential care workers in the course of conflicts with their charges.

THE POWER FACTOR

A major component in the residential care worker's intimate definition of a situation is his evaluation of the resources of the youths with whom he shares or is about to share that situation. He needs to do this in order to compare their power with his and thus evaluate his chances of imposing his definition of the situation on the encounter developing between them.

From the ethnographic materials gathered, it emerges that in their interactions, both residential care workers and their charges make use of their power—overt, covert, and semi-covert, whether in a veiled or an open, offensive manner.[10] How this is done certainly stems from personality traits and cultural patterns, but it is also largely contingent on the circumstances of the interaction. The power on both sides creates conditions of mutual dependence.

The Power of the Youth

The power of the youth appears to derive from two main sources. One source is their numbers. While the residential care worker is usually alone in the situation, a group of youths can organize to oppose his position. Werthman (1963), dealing with teacher-student interaction, shows how this kind of process occurs when students suspect that a teacher has been unfair to them or to some of them. A similar description is given by a residential care worker:

> *Benny*: A few weeks ago a young and very devoted madrich left—of his own free will. The source of his trouble was that his charges felt that he was not being fair to some of them. What did he actually do? The kids felt that there were some he talked to more, gave them more of his time. I know that he had good educational reasons for this. There are some kids who objectively need more attention. But the kids didn't buy that and saw it as discrimination. They formed a coalition against him; he tried to explain but it didn't help. A social worker they trust tried to intervene, but that didn't help much either. They decided he wasn't fair and showed their hostility to him in dozens of little ways, sometimes just by sulking, until he just couldn't stand it and left.
>
> It's not a question of whether you are fair or not; what counts is what the kids think of you. When it comes to things like that, there are a lot of them and just one of you.

In most of the residential care workers' descriptions of hurt, especially hurt to their colleagues, it is perceived and described as an act by a group (or "gang" or "Mafia"). The size of the group is not usually specified, and the term "hurt" is used in a generalized manner. The hurt is effective, either because the group is more powerful than the individual residential care worker or because the rejection by many–especially by the whole group–is an extremely painful insult.

> *Esther*: The regular em-bayit was on maternity leave and I was asked to replace her, but the kids decided that I didn't suit them and they boycotted me. Do you know what it is when 20 children don't just refuse to cooperate but refuse to exchange one word with you?

It appears, however, that being hurt by a group is not always worse than being hurt by an individual. A youth you are very fond of can sometimes hurt you more than several working together or even a whole group.

> *Henry*: A group is something vague and amorphous; individual people are real. When a whole group turns against me I can manage somehow. I try to understand the group dynamics that led to it and somehow we all calm down. It's much worse when it's one child, a child I've become attached to.
>
> There's that girl who came here after grade 6, when she was about 12. A real ugly duckling, full of anxieties and tics, untidy, wanting to be accepted by the other kids and being rejected by all of them, bullied by the bigger girls, hopeless at school. I think she was the first kid who actually brought out my paternal feelings, made me want to protect her, support her.
>
> As she grew up she even became quite pretty. I had every reason to believe I was important to her. At the beginning of this year, though, I began to notice that she was drifting away. In the dining room, for example, she began to sit far away from me. She stopped coming to various activities that I organized, such as a dancing group, and she loves dancing. One of her roommates even said to me half sarcastically: "What happened? Doesn't Sally love you any more?"
>
> I don't think it was an erotic love story, either on her side or mine. But we had become attached, and one fine day it all came to an end. I noticed that she was becoming closer to the em-bayit and I actually became jealous.
>
> A week ago, I happened to ask her to bring some of the group members to the clubroom. She looked down her nose at me and said, "Sorry, I'm not your servant," and she walked away. I felt betrayed. I felt worthless and redundant.

Felix: When a whole group drives me crazy, somehow I survive. But when one child who is a leader in the group shows hostility, I simply can't stand it.

The second source of the youths' power, apart from sheer numbers, is the residential care worker's dependence on their cooperation.

Gad: You face 20 kids or more, all of 12, 13 years old. Babies. But they have a common will. The fact that you are a sensible and responsible adult doesn't mean much.

Last year I found myself in this situation: A week earlier I had organized a terrific Sabbath celebration with them. The entire home, staff and kids, praised us. The group that was supposed to prepare the celebration the following week had a problem; their "star" singer was sick or something. I thought that after our previous success, this would be a good chance to shine again. That evening I brought up the subject. I pointed out the advantages and opportunities. Suddenly I felt that they were not with me at all. One of the leaders muttered: "We worked our butts off last week. Can't they organize their own evening? It's their problem. Don't dump it on us."

I looked around me. They were my group, and I would have liked them to comply with a reasonable request. But within a few seconds I realized that I didn't stand a chance against the solid will of the group.

As far as the residential care worker is concerned, the absence of cooperation means obstruction of his work, even if the failure to cooperate results from a chance set of circumstances and is not a deliberate act against the worker or experienced as such. In many circumstances the young people do not have to cooperate (e.g., there is no obligation for them to take an active part in the group discussions; generally, their physical presence is sufficient). Lack of cooperation with the residential care worker may be acceptable inactivity, and its very legitimacy enhances the power of the youth. The residential care worker usually has no practical possibility of attacking "legitimate" behavior.

The residential care worker is thus largely dependent on the good will of his charges: when they agree to cooperate, the worker accomplishes his work in a given situation. If for some reason they do not, and the reason could be intentional on their part or not, the worker cannot really accuse them of anything.

Even stronger is the residential care worker's feeling of helplessness in the face of behavior that not only thwarts his objectives in a specific situation but hurts him personally, yet still, like lack of cooperation, remains within legitimate bounds, and is therefore unassailable. Examples of this are Goffman's (1961) "subversive irony" and "half-open, half-hidden impertinence"—gestures or words that cannot be proved as intending to insult the madrich even though all those present—the worker and the group—know that that is their precise intention (Denscombe, 1985).

The youths' power may hinder the workers' ability to supervise and control what happens in a situation, while the workers feel that they need to develop effective strategies of supervision based on their power. More precisely, this depends on their perception of their present power and their assessment of additional powers they can summon in the next stages of the interaction—both of these in relation to their assessment of the power of their charges. The power of the youth in care thus threatens the residential care workers and contributes to their feelings of vulnerability—which breeds discontent.

NOTES

6. The meaning of this concept in the educational context, particularly the teacher's definition of the situation, is discussed by Stebbins in his work on the meaning of academic performance (Stebbins, 1977) and classroom ethnography (Stebbins, 1981).

7. While the madrich is a male in most cases and the em-bayit is almost always a female, the term residential care worker applies to workers of both sexes. The masculine pronoun is used for the sake of simplicity and does not reflect any gender bias.

8. As has been noted above, the interviewees were residential care workers. The names given are fictitious.

9. This approach to the subjectivity of disruption guides researchers from various traditions. See, for example, Hargreaves, Hester, and Mellor (1975) and Tattum (1982).

10. On the centrality of power in interactions taking place in organizations, see, for example, Comstock (1982) and Pfeffer (1989).

Chapter 3

Who Hurts?

The young people living in residential care settings are usually considered to be "problem children." Although this is not an objective statement, it undoubtedly reflects broad intersubjective agreement. The subjects who share in it–the "definers" and those who are thus defined–often include screening and placement agents and members of the youths' communities and of neighboring communities as well as residential care experts. Sometimes members of the resident's family and the resident himself concur with this definition as well. Young people are generally referred to residential settings because they were identified as "problematic" in their previous environment.

The "problems" of these youngsters are often, in fact, euphemisms for deviance from social norms in one, two, or all three of the following domains: In the cognitive domain, they are sometimes described as having considerably lower intellectual and scholastic ability than their peers. They may be perceived as physically different, disabled, sick, or limited. But it is mainly in the affective domain that they are seen as different–maladjusted, disturbed, disruptive, and sometimes delinquent and violent.

It seems to be very rare for youth who are not considered "problematic" to be referred to residential settings merely because they come from broken or poverty-stricken families. The fact of their being identified as deviant or "problematic" has special significance in the way they are perceived by their caretakers, the residential care workers, who do not usually question the validity of the considerations that led to the youths' referral to the setting and often take them for granted. In the interviews, the residential care workers described their charges at great length, referring to their behavior, their prospects, and the reasons for their referral to

[Haworth co-indexing entry note]: "Who Hurts?" Arieli, Mordecai. Co-published simultaneously in *Child & Youth Services* (The Haworth Press, Inc.) Vol. 18, No. 2, 1997, pp. 33-45; and: *The Occupational Experience of Residential Child and Youth Care Workers: Caring and Its Discontents* (Mordecai Arieli) The Haworth Press, Inc., 1997, pp. 33-45. Single or multiple copies of this article are available for a fee from The Haworth Document Delivery Service [1-800-342-9678, 9:00 a.m. - 5:00 p.m. (EST). E-mail address: getinfo@haworth.com].

the residential setting, dwelling on those who disrupt their work, disturb them, and hurt them.

PERCEIVED CAUSES OF THE WORKERS' PAIN

The residential care workers impute the "problematic nature" of the youth who hurt them to various sources according to the approach they adopt. The three major approaches noticed in the interviews are discussed below.

1. Downward Displacement of Blame

According to the first approach (which seems to be the most prevalent), there are two major kinds of deviance: cognitive and affective. Cognitive deviance is perceived as either congenital or environmental ("nature" or "nurture"). Affective deviance may be seen as resulting from biological, physiological traits (hyperactivity, for example) or from psychological trauma. The source of physical deviance may be a congenital defect or accident.

On the face of it, congenital deviance is more serious than deviance rooted in the environment or socialization, but in point of fact, environmental deviance is often perceived as no less deterministically constraining. Mental retardation is not significantly more severe than environmental deprivation when the latter emerges at a crucial stage for cognitive development, and the resulting deficits are considered to be severe and irreversible.

> *Henry*: They cannot understand and conceptualize at age 12 because at a critical time in their lives, say at eighteen months, when they needed a great deal of verbal and other interaction, their mother was not there for them.

> *Flora*: The child-rearing patterns of their ethnic group did not encourage such interaction with their mothers.

Psychological disturbances arising from traumas of infancy are perceived as no less severe than biologically-rooted disturbances.

> *Isaac*: With psychotherapy it takes a lot of hard work–if it's at all possible–to break down difficulties that stem from the inhibitions, fixations, and traumas of the early stages of development.

In other words, the youth referred to a residential setting often brings with him problems whose chances of solution seem to be limited, in view of the deterministic attitude often held by the residential care workers concerning the sources and nature of the difficulties. This has two implications:

First, the "blame," or responsibility, for the youth's condition lies with the youth himself, since he bears within him the sources of his "problems." In this case, after unsuccessful attempts at rehabilitation, residential care workers can always resort to what Lacey (1970) calls "downward displacement of blame." This means putting the responsibility for the situation on the weakest link in the social system, namely, the youth himself.

> *Gretel*: I have done everything I can for the child; what else can I do? After all, as they explained in the course, his behavior stems from critical and irreversible deprivation.

Second, the youth is often perceived as primarily needing compensation rather than rehabilitation.

> *Jacob*: It's like in a car accident, when somebody loses his eyes. You can't do anything about it. You can't rehabilitate his eyesight. You can only compensate him. You can give him money. You can train him to do something that doesn't require sight. You cannot really restore his damaged faculties.

The residential care workers often expressed the view that the youths' difficulties in learning and adaptation, their referral to the residential setting, and their tendency to hurt residential care workers all come from one source: a characteristic inherent in the youth or in his social background. This is what accounts for their tendency to disrupt and hurt. They disturb because they are disturbed.

> *Shamoon*: Some of them are actually slightly psychotic, from birth or early childhood. What can I do with these? I can arrange for them to be admitted to a psychiatric hospital. They give them drugs. They come back quite woozy but nothing changes very much.

> *Ephraim*: Joel comes from a very problematic family: an alcoholic father and a mentally sick mother. One of our problems with him is that everyone here—and that includes me and the principal and even the supervisor—is afraid of his mother. Every time one of her children

is scolded even mildly, she phones and starts cursing and threatening the staff. Once, they say, she turned up at the setting and hit an em-bayit. If you can't work with the parents how can you expect to do anything with the children?

Leor: This is another boy from what they gently call one-parent families. It's almost always the child of an unmarried mother. And I can tell you from experience: those unmarried mothers are a big problem. It doesn't surprise me one bit that many of the most difficult, infuriating kids are the children of unmarried mothers.

Ken: They say his mother's a whore. We don't know about that. In fact, she looks all right. Maybe she's just a sort of tramp. She's an adult; it's her business. But with a mother like that, it's no wonder that he rejects every woman on the staff.

A residential care worker explains that socioeconomic and cultural background is "everything." Those of her charges who come from "good, cultured homes" are motivated and can study well and behave satisfactorily.

Hilla: Isn't that the way with youngsters who come from neglected backgrounds? We all know that every child undergoes a socialization process at home, and that's what determines his ability to benefit from his education.

Naphtali: These youngsters come from difficult families; their parents are damaged. In many families you see that there are no boundaries, no clear norms, no one knows what is allowed and what is forbidden.

Porat: The ones who frustrate me most are those from problem backgrounds. They come from homes that are weak, non-supportive families, and all kinds of other problems.

Ohad: Sometimes I sit at home and talk to myself. I hope I'm not going mad. I ask myself if they do it on purpose to hurt me or if they are just like that, just grew up like that with psychological, mental, and physical deprivation. They are psychologically damaged with neurotic symptoms, severe traumas.

That's what I have to cope with. And I really do want to help them, that's what I'm here for.

The workers often expressed disappointment that the youth do not respond to the influence of the mainstream culture to which they are exposed in the residential setting. The youths' attitude toward the established culture is sometimes one of alienation, cynicism, and contempt. Some of them identify the residential care workers with the mainstream and consider them to be its representatives, although that is often not the case and the workers do not attempt to bring them into the mainstream.

> *Reuben*: One painful incident was when the whole group went to a play at a theater in Tel Aviv. The tickets were numbered and we were not sitting together as a group. I was the only adult escort, contrary to the rule, but I wasn't worried. Perhaps I was too optimistic. As the play started I suddenly heard laughter and whistling from the back of the auditorium. It was our kids. They whistled every time a pretty actress came on stage. They laughed out loud, made crude comments and catcalls, and yelled to the actors. Things like, "Speak up!" "What?" "Did you forget the words?" After a few minutes, they started shouting in unison: "Money back! Money back! We want our money back!" I thought I'd die of shame.
>
> What should I do? Should I go over to them and try to get them out? Raise my voice to them from where I was sitting? The people near me were whispering, talking about the kids and their rudeness. Their remarks were peppered with things like "Uncivilized" and "It's their rotten upbringing!" Somebody even called for the show to be stopped.
>
> On the way back from the play I didn't say one word. I tried to understand. After all, some of them were in a kind of culture shock; they had heard of theater, imagined what it was, but this was their first visit to a theater. Perhaps their rude behavior was an expression of alienation, as if they said, "This is your culture, rich people all dressed up in fancy clothes, it's not ours. Your artsy European stuff doesn't mean a thing. It doesn't do anything for us. You snobs don't really want to share it with us."
>
> I was hurt, but in fact they hadn't hurt me directly; I was hurt because of the embarrassment and because of the message: it's your theater, not ours! It's not part of our world, and we won't sit there and pretend that we give a damn about what they're saying on the stage. If we come here we'll come to tease you and the rest of the people like you.

A prevalent ideology among educators sets goals such as identity formation, choice, and the ability to fulfill one's personal needs autonomously (Levy, 1993). Some residential care workers think this ideology is partially achieved in the settings where they work, but others express severe disappointment and the feeling that these ideas are "not always practical" in guiding their work. They frequently expressed disappointment with the "parasitic consumer culture," as one of them put it, through which the youth relate to them.

Ken: Sometimes I'm hurt because I have the feeling that in their eyes I am just there to supply their needs. I'm all right as long as I give them what they want, but I'm not worth much when I stop giving and start talking about values like the need for them to give, not just to receive, or the need for them to choose, to plan, to use initiative, and to take responsibility.

Ilana: The setting tries to compensate the youth for the neglect they suffered at home. Because of this idea, everything they ask for is treated as a basic need to be supplied at once. Whether it's things for school, like crayons or pencils, or whether it's clothing or whatever . . . It's not that I think we shouldn't give them. What frustrates me is that they don't appreciate the cost of anything, they take it all for granted. And that's why they don't take care of what they get. They know that if they lose or spoil their crayons we'll run and buy them new ones.

For example, three and a half months ago one of the boys in my group got a new schoolbag. Not two months had passed when he came to tell me it had disappeared and he needed a new one. I said that we would look for the old one first, perhaps he had mislaid it somewhere. He didn't really cooperate, just looked hastily in one or two places and repeated his demand for a new one. I was angry at this approach of "buy me and bring me"; I told him we would go to the storeroom and look for an old schoolbag. He refused adamantly and told me half-threateningly that if I didn't buy him a new one he would phone his parents and tell them he'd been going to school without a schoolbag for the last few days.

In the end I did buy him a new one. It's only this year that he began to attend regular classes and I didn't want him to miss any lessons. My partial solution to the problem was that he paid something out of his weekly allowance towards the new schoolbag. He couldn't refuse because I'm the one who gives out the money. So you could say he was forced to give; he certainly didn't show any sign of thinking that he should contribute to that purchase himself.

Somehow we fail to draw the line between responding to their de-
privations and turning them into "little parasites."

In the residential care workers' opinion it is the youths' problematic
backgrounds that breeds their tendency to disrupt, to hurt, and to sabotage.
The situation is sometimes described as beyond change.

Judy: I've long stopped thinking I have tools or magic powers to
influence or change the situation. The type of population that comes
to us is simply like that. All we can do is deal with the immediate
problems that rise to the surface. Patch up here and there. I definitely
don't believe it's possible to reform these girls and make them
change.

3. Upward Displacement of Blame

According to the second approach, the source of the residents' problems lies not in themselves, or not only in them, but in the macrosocial
order. Several of the workers subscribed to this view, some of them supporting both this and the previous approach.

This argument shifts the responsibility for his problematic nature from
the youth to the wider social order. In its essence this approach suggests
that youth from weak social groups are sometimes referred to schools,
classes or residential settings that will not help to improve their lot. The
credentials they eventually receive from these settings will not promote
their chances of significantly improving their position in society when
they "graduate" from the setting. It is not that the settings are deliberately
designed to allocate low status and humble social roles to their wards, but
they unintentionally limit the prospects of intergenerational mobility. In
other words, the fact that many youngsters in weak social groups do not
reach higher educational and social attainments than their parents is explained by the settings' tendency to act as agents of social reproduction
(Sarup, 1978; Collins, 1979).

It seems from several of the interviews that the definition "problematic" applied to youth in residential settings may be explained by tendencies
of social reproduction. This suggests that the social center uses selective
procedures with regard to the admission of young people from weak social
groups to normative educational frameworks by defining some of them as
"problematic." This definition functions to stabilize the existing social
order. To use Lacey's (1970) expression, this explanation of the problematic nature of youth in residential care is "upward displacement of
blame."

In these circumstances, the residential care worker struggling to cope with difficult charges in the residential setting does not need to claim that his difficulties stem from the deterministic nature of the youth's "problem." Instead, he can argue that his difficulties in caregiving are the result of the deterministic nature of the social structure. According to this approach, the youth's problem is not one of care. Its solution will not come through generating change in the individual resident, but by creating change in the macrosocial order. The residential care worker feels that his charges disrupt or hurt him because they are reluctant to cooperate with a voluntary or involuntary agent of a depriving system.

Tal: Sorry to sound so radical, but I've become convinced here that the existing social order is to blame. That's what causes these kids' disruptive behavior no less than their personalities and background.

Tal: We have one boy here who is particularly clever and cynical. He never misses a chance to grumble or openly hurt the staff. He's not satisfied with just not cooperating with anyone or anything; he likes to demonstrate to his friends and mainly to the staff that "nobody can do anything to me" and that he simply doesn't like the setting and doesn't give a damn.

A few months ago, before bedtime, I was talking to him and his roommates. He said some very nasty things about the setting, echoed by murmurs of agreement from his pals. I said to him: "You're quite grown up, so why do you stay here? It's not a closed institution. Why don't you just leave?" "Look," he said, "in the town where I come from, every kid I know is in school until he's 18 and goes into the army. Either he's at a regular high school or a residential school. I suppose I could go to work, but no one I know goes to work before the army. What do you think I am, a moron, to go to work at 16-and-a-half?

"They wouldn't even look at me at a regular high school, so I came here. They accepted me here. The food and the girls are ok, but that doesn't mean I have to like you. What are you doing for us, anyway? What happens to us when we leave? What qualifications do we get here? All we do is pass the time somehow till we get a qualification that isn't worth much outside.

I could have been working long ago in something I'm supposed to be learning here, but according to the rules I'm still a student, still supposed to be learning, and that's why I work here for nothing when I could be working in a garage outside for money."

At the same time, for some reason he said that he had nothing against the staff; we're ok, according to him. The problem is that he sees being with us for several years as a sheer waste of time."

> *Vardi*: Then she (the girl) said something like this. "I'm mean to you because I think that you are also responsible for us not having a chance here. It's not enough for you to say that the authorities won't let us take the college prep program and then shut up. The kids here don't feel that you fight for us. You don't go out of your way to help. You only do what's convenient—and that's not much. We're mean to the staff because it's you—not only the big boys downtown—who help the system waste our lives."

3. Life in Residential Settings and Secondary Labelling

According to the third approach the problem of youth in residential care settings usually grows—and is sometimes even created—during the time they spend at the residential setting itself. The emphasis here is not on traits the youths have carried with them from the day they were born, on problems stemming from their backgrounds, or on defects created by macrosocial processes, but rather on problems rooted in their interactions with others in the residential setting, particularly the residential care workers.

Lemert (1967) distinguishes between primary and secondary deviance. Primary deviance is spontaneous deviant behavior—behavior characteristic of us all as human beings. There is hardly anyone who does not occasionally find himself violating norms. Whatever the cause, as long as the deviances are not too frequent and not seen as a threat to society or to the deviant himself, society finds mild ways to deal with them. But sometimes they cannot be ignored, and then society publicly defines the deviant as "disruptive," "violent," "disturbed," "incapacitated," "backward," "culturally deprived," and so forth, thus giving him a label, a new social identity.

Thus, the deviant undergoes a process of labelling. When an individual is perceived to fit the image of a certain type of deviant and publicly labelled as such, he becomes the target of expectations that tend finally to fulfill themselves, culminating in his becoming a chronic deviant in his daily behavior. This is secondary deviance.

Young people in residential care are prone to secondary deviance. The youth is referred to the residential setting because welfare agencies and his teachers in the community are unable to cope with his problem in normative ways, but their decision to send him to residential care is an act that is apt to crystallize his deviance as secondary deviance. Referral to the residential setting is a public act involving the youth's parents, neighbors and friends. It may include the expectation that he will act in a way considered to be typical of youths sent to that kind of residential setting, young people who bear the label that he now bears.

Within the setting, the residential care worker sees no problem in the definition "problematic" attributed to his charges by his more "professional" colleagues in the screening and placement services (e.g., psychologists, social workers, educational counselors), who apparently often function as very significant others for the child's residential care workers. At the same time, in the powerful environment of the residential setting, the residential care worker is a significant adult, if not the most significant other, for the inmate. These circumstances are very conducive to the process of accepting the label and, with it, the expectation and intensification of deviant or disruptive behavior.

> *Vardi*: For about two years I thought that many of the things that kids in the group did were meant deliberately to hurt me. One day we spoke about it in some workshop and suddenly the penny dropped: perhaps they don't hurt and don't mean to hurt? Perhaps it's often only in my head? I must admit that it helped. It didn't solve all the problems, but it helped.
>
> We have one girl who's always smiling. You could see it as a mocking smile, and that's what I did for a long time. You could explain it as a kind of habit, perhaps a smile of embarrassment. For months all my dealings with her were unpleasant. I was her madrich and I had to deal with her, but I found it unpleasant, until it occurred to me that maybe her smile was not one of mockery but something else, perhaps a form of defense. It's hard for me to explain, but a few days after I decided to look at it that way, I felt her attitude toward me changing, that she was changing altogether. In a heart-to-heart talk that I finally had with her she hinted to me that something about me had made her feel uncomfortable in the past, but it had changed, and she didn't know why.

> *Uzzi*: At the beginning of the year we hold a series of meetings devoted to planning activities and administrative arrangements. Usually they also bring in a lecturer or two from outside to expand our knowledge on relevant questions. They call it "preparation days." The educational counselor usually brings the files of the new admissions and gives us relevant information about them and their backgrounds. We aren't given the complete picture, though, because it is considered unethical for us to know everything. Only the "hallowed" professionals, for some reason, are allowed to know more.

At the beginning of this year some of us suggested that it would be better if they didn't tell us anything about the new admissions. In our hearts we wanted to protest the fact that we are not considered worthy of knowing everything, but we didn't say that openly. Anyway, the idea was accepted. We could guess a lot about the new kids from their appearance and behavior, but we could not be sure of the facts and might make mistakes.

Well, that's what happened. There was a boy who was clean and tidy, quiet and withdrawn but unusually polite. Never raised his voice, was never cheeky or insulting to any of the staff. He also spoke better and seemed more refined than the others. There were times when I thought: there's something wrong here, this kid is here by mistake. I liked him very much. So did the others. At the end of term there was a parents' meeting, but a social worker from his town showed up instead of his parents. We told her that we were very pleased with him, and she looked astonished and happy at the same time. It appeared that our well-mannered boy had been diagnosed at the end of grade 6 as borderline retarded with an IQ of less than 80. He also had two police files for robbery. As for his family–don't even ask! Evidently it was good that we didn't know!

An issue that occupied many of the workers was the question of whether youths who hurt them or their colleagues are consistent in these behaviors. Some think that "there are no rules about this." Incidents of hurt of various kinds are random events that cannot be explained by clear, consistent principles. An "easy-going" youngster "is liable to go wild all of a sudden for no reason that is clear to us or to himself." There are not generally consistent groups of obedient and well-behaved youth. And if a youngster joins up with an unruly group or organizes one around himself, this is almost invariably temporary and the clique will break up when the situation changes.[11]

Some of the workers thought that episodes that are perceived as hurtful are sometimes not only random but trivial, with no intention to hurt. Some thought that most of the youth and most of the groups who behave in a hurtful manner did not always, or even usually, behave that way.

> *Kalia*: It depends very much on the worker's personality and experience, on the level of the group, and on the kids' background, gender, age, and how long they have been at the setting. Also on their mood. On a very hot day at eight in the evening when they are dead tired, you can't do anything with them. If you try to do something, they'll hit back at you without thinking twice about it.

Analysis of the interviews indicates that what occupies the workers most is who hurts, the meaning of the hurt for them, its motives, and trying to understand their charges' world that brings them, among other things, to those behaviors that lead to the discontent of their caregivers.

In summary, the analysis revealed three approaches. According to the first, the youth and his background carry within them the characteristics that lead to the hurtful behavior; according to the second, the youth's situation and his hurtful behavior reflect the macrosocial order and his protest against it; according to the third approach, the motives for hurting residential care workers are largely inherent in the nature of the interaction between caregivers and care receivers.

This third approach, which uses the labelling argument to explain the problematic nature of the inmates' behavior, differs from its two predecessors in that it allows neither downward displacement of blame ("the youth carries his problematic nature within him") nor upward displacement of blame ("the problems are rooted in the social structure"), but rather sees the interaction between the caregiver and the care receiver as the key to the creation, definition, development, or perpetuation of the "problem."

This perspective is less deterministic than the other two, since it does not assume a causal relation between the phenomena. The inmate acts as he does, not because of a problem inherent in him or because of the impact of macrosocial forces, but in accordance with his caregivers' expectations. Expectations are something that can be influenced and changed. In other words, one of the advantages of the labelling approach is its intrinsic optimism. It is possible to improve the youth's situation by enhancing the worker's awareness of the powerful impact he has in labelling the youth and in the effect of his expectations on the young person.

In the field of schooling, there is fairly impressive evidence showing that teachers who direct positive expectations toward their pupils encourage them and help to develop their thinking and learning ability. In the field of residential group care, it seems highly likely that residential care workers who believe in their charges' ability to change and who express positive expectations in this direction can help them to change in those aspects which are considered "problematic" (Beker & Feuerstein, 1991; Wolins, 1969).

NOTE

11. The question of the continued and stable existence of subcultures among youth has been studied extensively in the world of the school. See, for example, Hammersley and Turner's (1980) theoretical review, in which they present in detail the views of Wakeford (1969), Lacey (1970), Woods (1979), and others who claim in different ways the continued and steady existence of subcultures in the classroom. These subcultures support, reject or hold some other consistent

attitude toward the teachers. In contrast, Hammersley and Turner (1980) also review the approach of Furlong (1976) regarding "interaction sets" in the classroom. These are presented as temporary and as stemming from shared definitions of situations and similar but passing interests of some of the students who joined together by chance. For a discussion of the issue in the residential context, see Arieli (1989), Lambert, Bullock, and Millham (1973), and Polsky (1962).

Chapter 4

Who Is Hurt?

The external evidence of hurt, based on observation, is diverse, from silence and withdrawal to noisy outbursts. The interviews focused partly on the experience of hurt, with many of those interviewed claiming that this experience is common among residential care workers but that it does not characterize them personally. Residential care workers feel hurt because they perceive their charges as hurting them, deliberately or otherwise.

Why do residential care workers tend to be hurt? What happens in their experience that causes the feeling of hurt? In the opinion of the interviewees, youth reject or hurt primarily those workers who are "deviance provocative." This is not a phrase they used, but a concept suggested by Hargreaves, Hester, and Mellor (1975) to describe experiences largely similar to those of residential care workers. These researchers argue that "deviance provocative teachers" are those who think "deviant" students act the way they do because it is their nature. Thus, their approach to these students is "provocative." They "attack" the "deviants"; they are quick to reproach them and to threaten them with punishment.

Their opposite numbers, characterized by the same researchers as "deviance insulative" teachers, believe that their students are basically good and that "deviance" is the result of circumstances and, therefore, can be modified. Their optimistic approach to "deviant" students pacifies them and prevents repeated incidents of deviance. As some of the workers put it:

> *Lea*: I think the group worker who is frustrated is one who is strict, impatient, and inflexible. She thinks the kids are like that by nature and there's not much you can do with them.

[Haworth co-indexing entry note]: "Who Is Hurt?" Arieli, Mordecai. Co-published simultaneously in *Child & Youth Services* (The Haworth Press, Inc.) Vol. 18, No. 2, 1997, pp. 47-60; and: *The Occupational Experience of Residential Child and Youth Care Workers: Caring and Its Discontents* (Mordecai Arieli) The Haworth Press, Inc., 1997, pp. 47-60. Single or multiple copies of this article are available for a fee from The Haworth Document Delivery Service [1-800-342-9678, 9:00 a.m. - 5:00 p.m. (EST). E-mail address: getinfo@haworth.com].

47

Yehuda: In time you learn that it's not so important what your co-workers say about the kids. There's often a big difference between what they say and what they think. A worker may talk as if she believes the kids can change, that the condition is the result of circumstances and it's all reversible, but in moments of stress her true feelings come out and she says that's the way they are and that's how they'll stay. And some are just the opposite. You think they're very negative about the kids' prospects of changing, but suddenly at some staff meeting, you find they really believe in the kids or in a particular one and insist on giving him another chance.

It depends very much what kind of script the worker has in his head, whether he believes in them or not. It's harder to change the script in the worker's head than to change the youngsters. And they grasp this long before we do. A girl once said to me, talking about the "liberal" George, "As far as he's concerned I'm finished, so why shouldn't I bug him a bit? No wonder he feels hurt. He's not like Sam, who cracks nasty jokes about us but everyone knows that he's really on our side, believes in us and all that . . . "

THE "INVESTMENT" FACTOR

Residential care workers think that the feeling of hurt is connected with their investment in their role: those who invest a great deal or very little tend to feel more hurt than those whose investment in their work is more moderate.

High Rollers

Those who invest a lot feel that much of their effort is wasted and tend to interpret their charges' behavior as rejection and hostility.

Porat: I think a person who puts a lot into his work feels more frustrated, because he expects more and then he feels that the kids reject him. He comes up against the dull reality and feels disappointed. I think the rule is, the more you put into your work the more disappointed you'll be.

Sometimes a group worker who is very involved tries to establish deep and meaningful ties with all his charges, a project that is doomed to failure and disappointment, especially in Israeli residential settings, where two residential care workers (a madrich and an em-bayit) are in charge of a group of perhaps 30-40 youths.

> *Daniella*: Those who think they can like everybody get hurt. . . . You can't get on equally well with 35 kids.

As has been noted, residential care workers tend to try to maintain close contact with their charges over long periods of time; they feel hurt when a young person they are close to decides, for reasons of his or her own, to "desert" them.

> *Zvika*: I was very hurt. After two years of building up a relationship of trust and mutual respect, the kid began to show signs of weakening and wanting to break this bond. I understand that it's like parents' love for their children, love that ends in separation. But that doesn't make it any easier.

Sometimes a residential care worker's devotion to his work arouses stress among his colleagues: he establishes standards they are not prepared to live up to.

> *Porat*: Sometimes there are problems with other staff members—workers who feel that you threaten their status by being too devoted to your work. A worker who is active and resourceful is a threat to one who is sleepy and lazy . . .

Occasionally this feeling is imputed to them by the "devoted" worker even though his colleagues do not feel it.

> *Leor*: That one always feels that the others want to push her out of the setting because she works too hard and the others are afraid they'll be expected to do the same. That's total bullshit. It's all in her head. I don't think she puts more into her work than the others. Anyway, nobody makes those comparisons here. I hardly know what she does and I certainly don't know exactly how hard she works.

Low Ballers

The ones who invest very little in their work are those who are detached, alienated, and have a low sense of commitment. They also tend to feel that the youth hurt them a lot, either because of their own guilt feelings or because they feel excluded by the environment.

Mirit: To him work is just a source of income. He doesn't relate personally. The kids sense it and they're hostile. One day they'll really go after him.

Zvika: A "cold" worker works in a technical way. He shows no warmth or affection, so his charges don't like him. They feel anger and distrust toward him. It's not surprising that they sometimes hurt him.

Reuben: There are some workers who can't or don't want to form strong ties with the kids in their group, so the kids don't give a damn about what they say and give them a hard time. Then the worker complains about being rejected and not being listened to.

"UNFAIR" RESIDENTIAL CARE WORKERS

Interviewees reported that their charges often hurt residential care workers who they think are unfair to them or their friends.

Tal: I come from one of those little towns in the Negev (the sparsely populated desert region in the south of Israel). This year for the first time, we admitted some youngsters from my home town, two boys and three girls. I know two or three of the families. In the middle of the first term, there was a big party there to celebrate the 45th anniversary of its founding. The director here received a letter from the school there asking that the five kids and myself be released for this special event. Permission was granted, and off we went for the day.

When I got back, it turned out that while I was gone, four of the kids in my group had formed a clique demanding special leave for them, too, to go to the wedding of a neighbor in their town. I sensed that I was in trouble, and I promised to take up the matter with the directors and recommend it, but permission was refused. A neighbor's wedding, they explained, is not an event that justifies special leave. I tried again, but it was no use. In the group they said it wasn't fair and stuck to the argument that if I had really tried, it would have worked out, that I had put my town above theirs and given preference to the kids from my home town.

I heard them bad-mouthing my town behind my back, using words like discrimination and stronger expressions. The boycott spread to the whole group. They believed I had been unfair. I had no choice but to ask my boss to come and explain the procedures and talk about what had actually happened. It was very embarrassing for me. He came the same evening, explained things, and tried to calm them down. At first it did not seem to help very much, and for several weeks I was still "unfair," but gradually it seemed to die down.

"WEAK" RESIDENTIAL CARE WORKERS

Residential care workers think that those who are hurt most often are not the "provocative" ones or those who "invest" too much or too little in their work, or even the ones who are considered unfair, but those who are seen by the charges as weak. Which residential care workers, in their colleagues' opinion, are regarded as weak by their charges?

The Residential Care Worker Who Cannot Control His Charges

The youth are impatient towards residential care workers who fail in a central aspect of their role: control of their charges. The interviewees also tended, explicitly or implicitly, to justify the hurting of a worker who is unable to exert authority.

> *Porat*: I think the worker who is more frustrated than others is the one who doesn't display authority and common sense. His charges see a character who cannot give them anything and lacks knowledge and the ability to relate to them. And one who only uses force is not respected; they lose all desire to cooperate with him. A person like that will be listened to less.

> *Claire*: I remember one worker who had a heart of gold. He came here full of good intentions and worked for about a year. But every time there was violence towards him, say a kid threw a stone or threw food in his direction in the kitchen, he would take it personally and run to the office. I kept encouraging him and told him that the kids were testing him to see how he would react. If they saw him running away, they would go on doing those things. He should show them that he's the boss . . .

Ball (1980), Beynon (1984; 1985) and others describe how the class tests or "susses out" [often with hisses that sound like the word] a new teacher who arrives at the school or class at the beginning of the year. They attempt to evaluate his strengths: his ability to impose his definition of the situation and his knowledge of the codes in the culture of the setting and the youth culture. Some of our interviewees described such early encounters as critical for their careers in the long term:

> *Daniella*: They would smoke in their rooms or in the clubroom, and others went even further and smoked outside my room to test me and see what I would do to them.

> *Ken*: In almost every case they got the better of me because I really didn't feel that I had the strength to fight them and I felt that I was much weaker than they were.

> *Isaac*: A new worker who comes to work has to face a lot of testing and provocation.

> *Naphtali*: Our kids are very quick to grasp an adult's weak points. Then they devise more and more tests for him. Some of them can be quite tough . . .

New residential care workers, more than veteran ones, feel they are emotionally, morally, or otherwise incapable of scolding a youngster or expressing straightforward anger at him.[12]

> *Hilla*: I just can't do it. It's not that I'm such a refined, tolerant person. It's an old weakness of mine, a destructive personality trait . . .

The Worker's Status and Prestige in the Organization

Residential care workers sense that their charges are well aware of the social structure of the staff community and the organizational structure of the residential setting, and that they tend to reject workers who do not enjoy high status and prestige in these frameworks.

> *Reuben*: I also think there's a connection between the status of the madrich or em-bayit on the staff and their frustration with their charges and their work. A madrich whose status is high among the adults is respected by the youngsters as a person with authority; he is more significant for them. If his status among the staff is not high, his charges tend to give him more trouble and to hurt him.

> *Felix*: We have a laundry worker, a woman who really puts her heart into her work, and it really hurts her that the kids mock her and tease

her. She sometimes comes to me to complain about one of my kids harassing her. I think they hurt her just because she doesn't have the power or status of a residential care worker.

Occupational Role and Private Life: Blurring of the Boundaries

Interviewees say that carers become more vulnerable to their charges' behavior in "total institutions" (in the Goffmanian sense; Goffman, 1961), where there is little geographical separation– even for the staff–between work, sleep, and play. In relatively closed settings, somewhat isolated from the outside community, when the boundaries between their private lives and their occupational roles become blurred, the workers' vulnerability increases.

Batya: At first I stuck around the cottage all the time. No more. Now I leave my troubles there and go home without even reflecting on them.

Ephriam: Some of the workers–I just don't know how they go on working in the setting and how their frustrations don't ruin their private lives. I definitely separate my work life from my private life, although I live on the grounds.

Abigail: A worker who is frustrated is one who doesn't know how to separate his work from his private life and takes all his aches and pains home with him. I think this has nothing to do with experience or age. It's that type of personality that can't keep boundaries.
There's someone like that at our place. She takes everything to heart, goes around scowling all the time, and acts as if this place is her whole world. She never goes home on time but always leaves at least an hour or two later.

The unmarried worker. For a single worker, without a family, it is even harder to separate his private life from his work.

Mansur: I think the worker who is more likely to become desperate is the young single person. If a worker lives here with his family, this is his home, but for someone who's not married it's not really home. For example, if I see a kid throwing garbage on the grass I tell him he's dirtying my home, because he really is. It's not a temporary room or apartment but a home in the full sense of the word . . .

. . . He has no home to go back to, even in the setting. Even settings that are not far from the city are somehow distant. So the staff live in the residential setting. You go a few hundred yards and you're home. If you have a family it's different, but it's hard for a bachelor in a residential setting. You feel embarrassed to start a relationship or fool around with a co-worker who lives nearby. It's not actually forbidden, but there is an unwritten rule that prevents you from seeming to behave too loosely inside the setting.

So you have to travel a long way to have a life of your own. Some bachelors do that. Others, especially the older ones, don't leave the setting. In the end their charges are the only family they have—a family that changes every few years, and leaves you no private life and no emotional security.

Batya: There are people here who don't separate their private lives from their work. If a person has no friends outside the setting and no other occupation, then clearly his work becomes his whole world. Even if he's still in school, he thinks about this place all the time, and he's more sensitive to everything that happens here. A person who doesn't separate his work from the rest of his life can easily sink into this. And people like that are naturally more vulnerable.

Cultural Distance

Some interviewees said that new immigrant residential care workers are more likely to be hurt. The residential education and care system in Israel seeks to employ new immigrant residential care workers because residential settings are perceived as a major tool for helping immigrant youth in their transition to the Israeli culture.

In the 1990s, Israel has been a major target for Jewish emigrants from the former Soviet Union and Ethiopia. To facilitate the process of cultural transition, some residential frameworks have sought to recruit some of their workers among immigrants from the same countries, although they may work with young people from elsewhere (including native Israelis) as well. Those who have not yet entirely resolved their own adaptation and absorption problems may have the most difficulty.

Ephraim: I think the worker who is hurt more than others is the one who is furthest from the kids in terms of personal and cultural background. I don't mean that a group worker has to come from a culturally deprived neighborhood, but the worker and his charges should have something in common. He should not be someone they see as a representative of the law, the establishment, the "other" culture, always preaching to them about discipline and order. There are workers like that, and I think the kids simply bug them and bad-mouth them, giving them nicknames like "whitebread."

Clara: When I began to work with these youngsters it was very hard for me. I come from Morocco, where the atmosphere was completely different. I never dared to raise my voice to my parents or teachers, let alone swear at them . . .

Gender

Almost all the interviewees, both men and women, think that women in residential settings are hurt more than men, for two main reasons. First, there are some who believe that women everywhere, by their nature, tend to be hurt more than men.

Jacob: I think female workers are more frustrated than males because they are weaker and more vulnerable.

Second, many residential care workers think that the influence of their culture of origin leads many of the youth to see women as more convenient victims.

Ilana: I think the female workers are more frustrated because the attitude the kids brought with them is that women are weaker and rank lower than men in society, so it is easier to take out their aggressions on them.

MODERATING AND DENYING PAIN

Many of the residential care workers spoke freely and animatedly in the interview, some of them even with agitation. Discussing teachers, Cole and Walker (1989) note that teachers are prepared to sit for hours with sympathetic listeners and "ventilate." Here, too, there is great similarity between teachers and residential care workers.

Some of the residential workers referred to the opportunity to deal with the subject of hurt as "tension release," a "cleansing," even a "therapeutic" experience. However, the hurt to the individual residential care workers themselves, not to the group or to a colleague, is not an experience they mention easily. Most of the interviewees have developed mechanisms for moderating and alleviating the pain or denying it as something they have experienced personally.[13]

You Don't Talk About It

Residential care workers are ambivalent about sharing their problems with others. On the one hand, they want to talk about their pain; there are some who choose to take part in support groups and workshops designed to help to ease the strain of their work. However, the residential care workers we interviewed quoted more examples of colleagues than of themselves, among other things because "It's not worth talking about it."

> *Henry:* Some of the staff members who live here are the adults who have been closest to me in the last few years. There are one or two I speak with about everything: health, money, future plans, and so on. But you don't talk about what you feel here at work; that's taboo. I think people are scared to expose themselves in that way so as not to show weakness, because in a way we are in competition.
>
> There's also the question of the bosses. We don't want them to know exactly what goes on in our work with the kids. Thank goodness, most of the work is done out of the sight of the bosses and away from the hearing of all kinds of professional counselors. Even so, if you talk about your problems to other people, even your best friends, you take a chance that they will get to know something you don't want them to know . . . in these things it's better to keep quiet. It doesn't pay to show that you are weak or hurt.

Not Me–Others

From the reports of the interviews it emerges that most of the interviewees spoke in generalized terms or they related episodes combining hurt to themselves and to their colleagues. Some interviewees did refer mainly to their own hurt, but most preferred to discuss hurt to residential care workers as a general phenomenon, illustrating it with incidents that had happened to their friends. Some of the interviewees were aware that they might be underestimating the hurt by displacement of the hurtful incident and the pain it had caused to another individual or to the group.

> *Felix:* You want to know what happens to workers in general, not to me personally, right? So what difference does it make to you if I give

you general information or information about other people? And honestly, I'm an old hand, I don't get involved in any big dramas. I manage quite well, as a matter of fact. The problem is with some of the others.

Flora: Perhaps you're right and I'm avoiding or suppressing my problems a little. It's easier to talk about somebody else's problems. Apart from that, at the moment I really can't recall even one incident that happened to me personally.

Daniella: Nobody has hurt me personally the whole time I've been here. I can remember cases of other workers being hurt.

Not Now–Then

Displacement of the time of the hurt to the past, to the beginning of their careers in group care when they were "naive and inexperienced," is another common way of alleviating the pain and emphasizing the experience they have accumulated since then and the control they have acquired:

Leor: The main frustrating incidents I can remember are from my early days working here. I remember in the "group discussions"–meetings we have when the kids come back from school to talk about the events of the day, like problems of discipline, changes in work rotas, and on–they just didn't listen to me. A lot of them didn't even bother to come; some of them came and grumbled. I felt like I was talking to the wall. I really dreaded those meetings. I preferred to start working an hour later just to avoid facing that situation.

Gretel: When I first started in the setting I was sure that the kids disturbed only me, and that all the other workers, even the new ones, didn't have any trouble. I was too embarrassed to ask the other workers or to consult our supervisor.

Leah: Last year I worked on myself to become less irritable and not get angry and shout at the kids all the time. This year I'm more relaxed, I take things easier, and I don't get hurt so much.

Not All of Them–Just One Deviant

Being hurt by one individual may sometimes be no less painful than being hurt by the group. But an individual who hurts can be perceived as deviant, and the act of a deviant does not represent the general attitude towards the person hurt. Thus, the idea of deviance inherent in an individual serves the residential care workers as another pain-relieving mechanism.

> *Uzzi*: There must be some sociological rule that there has to be at least one deviant in every group of 15 to 20 boys and girls. I've been in this business for eleven years, and every year I've had one or two, at most three of those. You know, problematic, deviant. It's not just that *I* think they're deviant. There's nobody here who thinks otherwise–among the staff or the kids. Say I'm busy with the group 48 hours a week, I'll spend at least 24 hours on them and the other 24 on all the rest. Sometimes I pray that they'll leave, or at least leave my group. But the thing is, they need us more than the others. Apart from that, as soon as they leave, some other kids will take their place as the deviants or I'll get a new "supply" of deviants from outside.
>
> It depends to some extent on the type of deviance, but most of them never really change. There are some who are passive and quiet. Their problem is that they hardly do anything, they're "barely alive." If you wanted to, you could ignore them and their problems. But most of the deviants are troublemakers. No matter what you do for them, they'll bug you, hurt you, insult you. It's lucky they're not the majority.

All's Well That Ends Well

Some of the pain is removed when the residential care worker can state that even if he was hurt at the beginning of an incident, he got the upper hand in the end. The worker feels that in the end he "reached" his charges, or "beat" them and managed to exert his authority. Therefore, he organizes events so that in the end he will restore the positive impressions and, despite the initial humiliation, confirm his professional image in his own sight and in the sight of others.

> *Hilla*: After that they didn't cooperate with me for a few days. Never mind. I won't say it didn't bother me, but I know from experience that in the end they always look for a way to make up with me. Sometimes it's worth suffering for a week, hoping that they'll understand in the end, to have that wonderful experience when they come back to you–not because you are strong but because they realize you were right, and because you mean a lot to them.

Multiple Strategies

Some residential care workers, in describing experiences of hurt, used all four strategies for softening the negative impression, whether for themselves or for their interlocutors. First, they connected the incident not only with themselves but with others as well; second, they located the hurtful incident in the early stages of their career; third, they attributed the hurtful behavior to an individual and not to the group; fourth, they ended the story with an account of "victory."

Dan: Five years ago I had a boy in my group who smoked grass. He was sixteen years old, and he had a very tough background. He came from a family with four other children, and his parents had rejected him; they said he terrorized them and his younger brothers and sisters and they couldn't stand it. To throw him out of the setting would have been like putting him out on the street. I must say that he behaved ok with me. He wasn't a saint, but we had unspoken agreements that worked quite well.

With anybody who replaced me it was terrible, especially his mockery. Once he offered a young woman worker a puff of a joint in front of some of his friends. When we didn't react severely the woman left. He knew there was not much we could do. One day he decided for some reason to have a public contest with me to see who was stronger. During the evening program he suddenly started singing when I began to speak. At first I laughed, then I saw that he was determined to show everybody who was the boss here. Every time I opened my mouth to speak he burst into song.

We had just learned about the Russian educator, Makarenko. He had a pupil like that and one day, perhaps without thinking too much about it at first, he decided to ignore all the pedagogic rules and give the boy who was challenging him a resounding slap in the face. I don't know where I got the strength and the courage to do it, but the next time I started to speak and he broke into song I walked over to him, looked him straight in the face and gave him a resounding slap on the left cheek, a Makarenko slap . . .

There was a frozen silence. You could have cut the air with a knife. It didn't make that boy a reformed character, but after that we treated each other with respect . . .

CONCLUSION

Thus we see that most residential care workers experience hurt at some stage in their work. In the workers' opinion, those who exercise power in a way their charges feel is unfair are often hurt. On the other hand, they also mention power and status in the organization and the ability to demonstrate power as vital assets in their work.

Indeed, the largest group who are hurt, according to their colleagues—and one that includes at some stage or another almost every one of them—is the group of "weak" residential care workers—those who have trouble exerting authority, who lack experience in residential care or are unfamiliar with the dominant culture, those whose only home and sole occupation is the setting, and women residential care workers.

We see also that residential care workers who are hurt develop mechanisms to alleviate the pain. First of all, silence: "We don't talk about it." In addition, we observed three forms of displacement used by residential care workers in reporting incidents: "Not me, other people"; "Not now, then"; and "Not all of them, only one." Another pain-alleviating mechanism that we discerned concerns the actual reporting: "All's well that ends well."

NOTES

12. On difficulty in expressing anger at students, see Pollard (1985).

13. The development of mechanisms for alleviating the pain of hurt is a coping strategy. Nevertheless, it seems better to discuss this development here, in the chapter dealing with the workers' perception of their situation, rather than in the chapter devoted to coping (Chapter 6), because the adoption of these mechanisms affects the workers' definition of their situation in the residential settings.

Chapter 5

What Hurts?

Lambert, Bullock and Millham (1973) describe the characteristics of what they call "informal social systems" of youth in residential care settings in terms of their relationship to the "formal social system," that is, the management and staff. In their study they found that the youth often develop informal systems that support, manipulate, openly reject, or are indifferent to the formal social system. These informal systems frequently function to keep the youth as far away as possible from the formal system and from the residential care workers.

RESPONSES TO THE FORMAL SOCIAL SYSTEM

Lacey (1975) suggests that the first two forms of relationship to the formal social system listed above–support and manipulation–characterize students in teacher education programs as well. There are some who support the formal system or–in Lacey's words, their relationship to the members of the formal order, those who are involved in their training, is one of "internalized compliance"–but sometimes the motives for seemingly supportive relationships are manipulative, a stance described by Lacey as "strategic compliance."

The Supportive-Internalizing Orientation

Our residential care worker interviewees described four orientations. The first, the supportive-internalizing orientation, is expressed in behavior

[Haworth co-indexing entry note]: "What Hurts?" Arieli, Mordecai. Co-published simultaneously in *Child & Youth Services* (The Haworth Press, Inc.) Vol. 18, No. 2, 1997, pp. 61-73; and: *The Occupational Experience of Residential Child and Youth Care Workers: Caring and Its Discontents* (Mordecai Arieli) The Haworth Press, Inc. 1997, pp. 61-73. Single or multiple copies of this article are available for a fee from The Haworth Document Delivery Service [1-800-342-9678, 9:00 a.m. - 5:00 p.m. (EST). E-mail address: getinfo@haworth.com].

61

characterized by conformity or over-conformity, which may embarrass the workers but never hurts them; on the contrary, they are pleased to see that their charges support them and internalize their and their colleagues' educational messages.

> *Kedem*: Nobody loves the flatterer, the one who repeats everything you say only louder and does everything you ask on the spot without hesitating. You suspect that he won't become a person with a fully-formed identity and self respect, but it's so easy to work with youngsters like that . . .
>
> We had a girl like that. She sensed that I wasn't too fond of her. One day she came to me and said, almost in tears, "Do you think I should be bitchy now and then?" "Yes," I said, without hesitating. For a few weeks she became a radical rebel. It amused me and the other kids, and she noticed that, but I didn't say anything. Gradually she found the balance and became cooperative again but did not overdo it like before.
>
> To emphasize her separation from me, she chose politics. I tend to be somewhat right of center. She became the chief spokesperson of the left, in fact the only one in my group. She says jokingly, but it always gets my goat, that as far as she's concerned, everything should belong to the workers and military action is never justified.

Strategic Compliance

Residential care workers are ambivalent toward manipulative youth, the ones who adopt an approach of strategic compliance, and are often hurt by their behavior. In point of fact, these youths "behave" similarly to the supportive ones, the internalizing compliants. But the latter fulfill the workers' expectations through identification, while the intentions of the former do not match their behavior. They "work the system," acting out of "secondary adjustment" to the total institution (Goffman, 1961). A long-term residential care worker in a not very prestigious religious residential school, many of whose students, for various reasons, do not come from religious homes, says sadly:

> *Benny*: At the beginning of the first year I explain the rules to them: "You have to observe the Sabbath, we don't eat non-kosher food, we pray three times a day, and the boys are to wear a skull-cap. The girls have to dress modestly; they must not wear slacks or mini-skirts." And they accept it; they follow the rules. During the three or four years they live and study here I rarely have any complaints about

them. But as soon as they finish school and get their certificates, while I'm still standing by the gate to say goodbye, right there in front of my eyes I see some of the boys take off their skull-caps and put them in their pockets and some of the girls open an extra button on their blouses . . .

In this chapter I shall mostly discuss the behaviors neither of internalized compliance nor strategic compliance but of those who openly reject the system or relate indifferently to it.

Indifference

Indifferent behaviors (such as passive behaviors or omissions, referring to what one does or does not do, respectively) can be divided into two groups: *legitimate* indifferent behaviors and *illegitimate* indifferent behaviors. Each of these will be discussed separately.

First, I will look at situations in which the worker's discontent is a result of the avoidance of cooperation with him. Residential care workers view such avoidance as undesirable but not "illegitimate" behavior. This refers to situations such as avoiding communication with the worker, withholding response to his therapeutic or consultative initiatives or pastoral care, not participating actively in group discussions, and disconnecting from what goes in such discussions.

Second, I will discuss the meaning of discontent as a response to non-performance of formal tasks, such as keeping to the daily schedule, going to school, keeping bedrooms clean and tidy, and taking one's turn at doing chores. Although not cleaning the dormitory and not taking part in discussions are both omissions, avoidance of communication with the residential care worker or withholding response to his consultative initiatives are not usually perceived as illegitimate offenses, but the failure to do chores or to get up in time for school are defined by the residential care workers as specific infringements of the rules, that is, illegitimate offenses.

Third, I will discuss the meanings of active behaviors that cause discontent and that residential care workers perceive as offenses—behaviors that, deliberately or otherwise, hinder the progress of their work.

Avoidance of Cooperation as Legitimate Omission

Most of the interviewees chose to tell us of their experiences with withdrawing behavior expressed through passive avoidance of cooperation with residential care workers. This can be described as legitimate non-cooperation. It is forbidden for the youth to disrupt, but it is legitimate not to take an active part in the group discussions; they are obliged to keep themselves and the dormitories clean and tidy, but they are not obliged to share their problems and worries with the residential care workers; they usually have to function in the formal school framework, but in the informal educational system after school hours they are free in most residential settings to cooperate or avoid cooperation with their residential care workers.

> *Gad*: I can't stand this passive resistance: I speak to them and they don't respond; I try to communicate and they seem to ignore me. No, they aren't openly cheeky, they just ignore me. In fact, I wish they would be cheeky, shout, and run wild. I can cope with rowdy behavior, but I can't cope with those silences.

> *Henry*: I'm hurt because I see myself somehow begging them to say something, not to leave my words in the air. I try to hide it, to pretend I don't care, that it isn't my problem. But they know I'm dependent on their response. Let's face it: my survival depends on them, not theirs on me.

Some of the interviewees think that the youth are aware that the objectives of the residential care setting are often the adult staff's objectives, not their objectives as adolescents, although the prevalent rhetoric describes them as the common objectives of the whole community of adults and youth.

> *Yehuda*: We act as if the youngsters joined the setting as voluntary members and therefore have to accept the rules and do as we say. But they know that their coming here was not exactly a free choice. They have to be here, but that doesn't necessarily make them feel good about it. They tell us so in all kinds of ways: "The rules here are your rules, not ours. Even when you act as if it's all democratic and equal, you really expect us to obey you in the end. So forgive us if we don't always feel like dancing to your tune."

A common situation, say interviewees, is that youth do not think they are in residential care settings to develop or be rehabilitated, but that it is simply "the lesser evil," the result of their life circumstances.

> *Vardi*: They are here because adults in their community think it is better than their broken home or the street. It's a solution for them, too, a comfortable and convenient environment. The food's not bad,

they have a decent room, various facilities, entertainment, and above all, kids their own age to hang out with.

The residential care setting is the main social environment of *all* its charges–those who identify with the objectives of the formal system and those who do not. Workers think that many of the youths believe it is best to humor them, especially those they consider to have more resources and power. According to this argument, the residents think they should try to give the workers the minimum they ask: to cooperate with them, at least ostensibly–that is, not to openly sabotage their role–and to let them "educate and care" even when their charges are not interested in this education and care.

However, the workers are not usually content with appearances but expect their charges to fulfill their role in the educational mission by actively taking part in situations which they, the residential care workers, generally initiate.

> *Dan*: I ask myself almost every day why it is so important for me to know every moment whether they are with me or not . . . But the urge is too strong for me, and I ask questions and try to get them to talk.

Sometimes non-cooperation is part of the youths' negotiations with the residential care worker over their varying definitions of the situation, negotiations that may end in a shared definition with which both sides can live comfortably. Even if the youth "disconnects," the residential care worker may prefer this to disruption (Reynolds, 1976), but such non-cooperation is more likely to be experienced as a crisis.

> *Tal*: When they are silent it makes me feel as if I don't exist. Sometimes they "do me a favor" by coming to the clubroom for a meeting, as if to say, "What are you complaining about? We're here, aren't we? So if you have something to say, say it."

Illegitimate Omissions

Educators tend to stress the importance of freedom of choice for the development and consolidation of an adolescent's identity in a residential care setting. The setting provides various options, but what enables the youth to develop his identity as an autonomous individual is not the existence of the options but the individual's right to choose among them and to decide on a course of action.[14] Several of the interviewees expressed this idea in various ways, revealing their identification with it and a wish to work in that context.

Asher: That's exactly what I believe; that's the way I'd like to work: to treat them like autonomous human beings, to let them choose, to stand by and intervene discreetly only when I feel they want me to. That's individuation the way they describe it in the textbooks; that's the educational process that allows every individual to reach self-actualization, to realize his inclinations and his freedom. It depends on us more than on them. It takes a lot of courage, but I believe that one day we will dare to work like that.

Kalia: Respect for the young person's decisions is not an empty slogan, but we abandon it again and again. Our charges, like us, are creatures of habit. They are in the habit [from before they came] of not getting up unless they feel like it, they are used to leaving a mess after themselves, they are used to being late. Time is not important to them. We try to help them build a different life, but again and again they let us down and we let them down.

A typical example is going to school in the morning. We have vehicles to take them to school, and they have to leave on time so we can drop them off at two or three schools. But one of the girls doesn't feel like getting up. At first you try to reason with her, but in the end, almost invariably, you lose your patience. You feel deep down that you know better than she does what's good for her. You raise your voice . . . and there you are, dictating her actions, and your pedagogic beliefs go out the window. I am not saying that those principles don't work, but they don't *always* work. The youngster is entrenched in his own habits much more deeply than you are entrenched in your pedagogic beliefs.

Thus, despite their pedagogic convictions, most of the residential care leaders and their staffs tend to see omissions connected with life routines as illegitimate. It is not possible to require the residents to maintain communication with the residential care worker (the absence of which is a legitimate omission), but it is possible to insist that they keep their rooms clean, do their homework, and keep to the schedule (all requirements where failure to comply would represent illegitimate omissions).

Claire: Until two years ago I used to get them off to school in the morning. The em-bayit had to wake them up and send them down to the dining room; I would keep order in the dining room and make sure all the busses left on time . . . Today I stay with them in the dining room and another worker sees to the transportation. I am with the kids during breakfast and I see the problems there: they don't clear their plates off the table, they arrive at the last minute and walk into the kitchen just when the bus is due to leave, and they get angry when I send them out. The whole business of kids missing school drives me crazy.

Leah: I organized a party on the evening of one of our holidays. The kids from the CIS [former Soviet Union] walked in as if they had been coerced into coming. The whole thing became a fiasco.

Nira: In the afternoon the kids have tea and a sandwich in the kitchen. Invariably, they leave the kitchen counter full of crumbs, jam, chocolate spread, whatever . . .

Routine chores comprise a major issue in the interactions between the residential care workers and the youth. All the youth are supposed to take turns doing cleaning chores in their living units. On the face of it, this is a simple organizational arrangement to ensure that their quarters will be clean and tidy. For the workers, however, these duties often represent their charges' attitude toward them.

Flora: A kid who is supposed to clean the dormitory corridors in the morning and avoids doing it is not just being irresponsible. He's telling me something. He's saying, "It's important to you, but I don't give a damn about it!"

Seeing these routine tasks done smoothly and on schedule is taken by the workers as evidence that their charges are "doing their duty"; expressions like "taking their duties seriously" reveal their view of these chores as one measure of the youths' level of functioning, acquiring good habits, and responding to the staff. Failure to perform such tasks is seen as negative feedback. Thus, the workers' overt concern with supervision of routine chores permits them to assess their effectiveness. They demand performance. If they receive it, they feel rewarded; if not, they become discontented.

Open Rejection–Active Hurting

Disruptions and hurt are not generally defined as such by the actors involved in creating them, the youth; they are the definitions held by the residential care workers in response to the actions (or inactions) of their charges. As noted above, the workers use the word "hurt" to refer to what they see as intentional behavior, rather than as behavior that is not deliberately intended to hurt them.

Residential care workers think that youth who openly reject them act as individuals or in small groups that are, they emphasize, typically transitory. That is, they emerge in certain situations and usually disappear shortly afterward. Furlong (1976) calls similar transitory situational groups of adolescents "interaction sets." In his view, these are not cohesive and consistent informal systems but generally temporary associations of students who define an evolving situation in a similar way. In the residential setting they make life difficult by behaving in an actively hurtful manner; they may disturb the residential care worker with laughter and open mockery, deliberately make a mess in their rooms and the dormitory buildings, or steal food from the kitchen for a midnight picnic.

Such rejecting interaction sets, characterized by hurtful behavior, often organize, say the workers, in the course of evening activities. In most Israeli residential settings, residential care workers hold evening meetings with their groups once or twice a week. These meetings, attendance at which is usually obligatory, have the paradoxical nature of an informal activity that formally requires the presence of all the group members. Sometimes these gatherings are devoted to a discussion of broader topical issues and sometimes to specific, practical matters concerning the group's life, such as planning a trip, a party, or volunteer work for the local community. These meetings have their origin in the earlier Israeli youth movements, which had considerable influence on the character of Israeli residential care settings.

This aspect of the program, with its ritual significance, is often considered a test of the residential care worker's leadership and competence. For the youth, the meetings provide an excellent opportunity to test or "suss out" a new worker. In many residential settings the evening meeting is regarded as the peak of the residential care worker's professional activity. Some residential care settings maintain a special pedagogic center that develops programs for evening activities for the residential care workers' use. On the other hand, some settings have abolished the evening meetings in recent years, mainly because of their formal nature, which some educators think is not compatible with the informal approach that is supposed to guide the evening activities of the group and the residential care worker.

It is almost impossible to describe hurtful acts that are considered as such by all residential care workers in all circumstances. What hurts one residential care worker does not hurt another. Behavior that the worker sees as hurtful in the evening gathering or at a particular time is not hurtful in a different activity or at another time. However, two acts that residential care workers almost universally defined as disruption or even mild hurt were nonattendance at the evening meetings and talking without the residential care worker's permission during the meetings. We will discuss these as common examples of illegitimate action.

> *Abigail*: I'm in charge of 17-year-olds in their last year of secondary school before joining the army. They're studying for their final exams. I prepared a session on army service, but when I arrived for the evening meeting I found I had no audience. They just hadn't bothered to come. One of them showed up and explained it to me: "Look, we'll be going in the army soon, and we already know all about it. It's a pity to waste the time when we could be studying for our exams." And others say, "If we have an hour to spare, it's better to see a show on TV. We have enough serious talks at school. Why should we waste time on things like that in the evening instead of relaxing?"

> *Tal*: I prepared a series of sessions on "decision making." It was a disaster. It took me a month and a half to prepare the stuff, which included personal decision making and collective decision making. I thought these things would grab them. But the response was a show of boredom, with kids leaving in the middle "to go to the bathroom" and not coming back.

Talking

Many of the workers who were interviewed revealed an ambivalent attitude towards talking without permission. None of them defined it as illegitimate behavior in all circumstances, nor did any of them say that the youth are entitled to talk whenever, however, and as much as they want to during the evening meetings. However, they differed in explaining their objections to talking and justifying their own and their colleagues' inclination to occupy most of the meeting with long monologues. They also differed in the importance they attached to the various explanations. Talking is, first of all, noise, especially when several people talk in loud voices all at the same time. Residential care workers said they could not physiologically or psychologically tolerate loud talking beyond a certain threshold.

Pedagogic Objection. A frequent explanation for the residential care workers' objections to the youths' talking during the evening meetings, and their justification for forbidding it, is that it detracts from the effectiveness of the activity. The workers have certain objectives that they wish to achieve, and they feel that when the youths speak without permission they are liable to distract their friends' attention from the subject of the discussion and thus obstruct the achievement of these objectives. This is how the workers expressed their fear that if the youth spoke spontaneously, even on the subject of the evening, they might irreparably deflect the planned and anticipated course of events.

The workers expect their charges to take part in discussions they conduct, often basing the meeting on such a discussion; for example, by questions and answers. Many of the youth are aware of this and act accordingly, either because of their tendency to respond to the worker's expectations or because the subject interests them. But in some of the discussions we observed there were youths who spoke spontaneously and, in the worker's opinion, they disrupted the course of events just by doing so.

This kind of disruption has two main forms, the most common being what Keddie (1971) describes as deviance from "the structure of relevance": during the discussion youths raise arguments that do not match what the residential care worker considers to be relevant to the subject being discussed or as "appropriate" ways of speaking in a discussion.

> *Daniella*: We were discussing the poverty of the tenants of a nearby senior citizens' home. The idea was that we would eventually do some volunteer work for them, but it was not on a practical level yet. The issue was the poverty of people, some of whom we actually knew. Then all of a sudden, Ruthie's high-pitched voice hushes us all. She insisted on telling us at that very moment about how her family was destitute before they immigrated to Israel. . . .
>
> Ruthie's a popular kid. Her mates didn't stop her, but some were uncomfortable, grinning in their embarrassment. It was obvious that her story was irrelevant to what we were discussing, but you have to be brave to try to stop Ruthie when she feels like talking. . . .

The second form is excessive or uncontrolled participation. The youths' behavior is sometimes defined as hurtful not because of deviance in its content, but because of the way the youth participate. They are "over-active" they speak to the point, but without waiting for permission.

> *Reuben*: This little guy, Pinchas, is an odd sort. He apparently knows a lot about religious, mysterious, and esoteric matters and enjoys showing off his knowledge about these things. I can raise any issue I consider suitable and Pinchas will say something religious about it . . . and at great length! I get frustrated. Other kids who want to say something get annoyed, too, but Pinchas goes on and on . . .

The residential care worker's interactions with his charges during the evening meeting can be classified into three types, based on who initiates the action and how it is received: sometimes the interaction is initiated by the residential care worker, sometimes by the youth and approved by the residential care worker, and sometimes by the youth and not approved by the residential care worker.

This last kind of talking without permission is discussed–in the school framework–by Jackson (1968), who presents the problem of coping with what he calls experiences of "immediacy."[15] The workers seek to follow a course of action they have planned, but often they are confronted with unexpected developments that compel them to adopt an alternative course of action immediately.

> *Tal*: Planning an evening meeting is a tedious activity, and then when you try to implement what you were planning, a guy raises an important angle you haven't thought about. You can either ignore him and get on with your pre planned agenda or you can relate to the unexpected new angle. I choose the second option; I ignore my preparations and improvise. At the end of the year I find that I haven't done most of the things I was planning to. Some of us here believe it's better that way, that "The kids know best what's worth discussing." I'm not so sure.

Residential care workers themselves wonder to what extent the prohibition they impose on speaking is designed to further educational objectives and to what extent it is designed to protect their original course of action for their own convenience.

Endangered control. None of the residential care workers we interviewed denied that the threat to their control is one of their motives for forbidding spontaneous speech. Speech is itself a tool of control in the evening meetings. Nevertheless, at the beginning of the interview many residential care workers tended to present their reaction to this threat as a pedagogic one and a response to the nuisance of noise. The worker's control in the residential setting is related to his status in the setting and in the community. Workers are sometimes afraid of the loss of control that may result from their charges' doubting or criticizing information transmitted to them during the group activities, or even debating or challenging this information.

Some residential care workers feel that their overall authority over the youth depends to some extent on their being perceived by the latter as epistemic authorities, that is, authorities in matters pertaining to knowledge (Raviv, Bar-Tal, & Peleg, 1990).

> *Tal*: At this age it is important for them to believe that I know best. They feel confused and disappointed when they realize that informa-

tion I gave them was inaccurate or that my judgment of things was wrong. This is often reflected in their immediate behavior toward me. I tell them many times that I am not an expert on anything. They understand it, but I doubt that they accept it.

Another aspect concerns talking as a challenge to the worker's authority and right to determine the order of the evening meetings, among them the order of speakers and actual permission to speak. The threat to his control of the group relates to the speaker's intention–the intention that the worker imputes to him–more than to the loudness and duration of the speech and the number of speakers.

Appearance of endangered control. These difficulties–the pedagogic objection to noise and the threat to the residential care worker's sense of control–are experienced as hurt in the situation of the evening activity. But the individual worker is also a member of the residential staff who feels the need to convince his colleagues and superiors that he is capable of youth care and education by the criteria that he thinks they use to evaluate his competence. One of the main criteria, in his opinion and apparently in theirs too, is his ability to control his group of charges.

The residential care workers and their superiors have limited access to knowledge about each individual worker's ability to control. The youth are directly exposed to that control and can, collectively, judge the relative competence of various workers, whereas the adults can gauge the individual's ability only indirectly through things the youngsters tell them about their colleagues or when a colleague turns to them for help. An apparently more commonly used indicator is the level of noise rising from the meeting room. The absence of loud talking or other noise by the youth is a clear sign of control.

Noise emitting from the meeting room is what Denscombe (1985) refers to as "publicly available knowledge." This provides, or so the residential care workers think, evidence of problems with control. Since their colleagues and superiors do not generally have direct reliable evidence of the workers' control over their charges in the group meetings, the workers endeavor to develop at least the appearance of control by forbidding speech.

Thus, residential care workers tend to object to their charges talking without permission during the evening meetings for various reasons, some of them congruent and some mutually exclusive. Talking without permission during these activities is a disruption to the residential care worker's work and sometimes to his feelings.

CONCLUSIONS

In chapters 3 to 5 we have reviewed the residential care workers' perceptions of situations in their group, specifically concerning the feeling of discontent many of them experienced in their interactions with the youth in their care. This review included descriptions and attempts to develop generalizations concerning the nature of the youth who "hurt" workers (chapter 3), the residential care workers who are particularly prone to being "hurt" (chapter 4), and the "hurting" actions (chapter 5). Most of the workers reported that they and their colleagues feel particularly hurt when their charges withhold their cooperation.

In the education and care conditions prevalent in recent decades, the youths' cooperation with their residential care worker is a necessary condition for the existence of every encounter between them. Cooperation is not a clear and uniform concept but a generalized name for what the residential care worker (like the teacher in the classroom) expects his charges to do or not do in their interactions with him.

Having located the residential care workers' definitions of the colleague who is hurt, we find that, rather than excluding those who are not mentioned, these definitions teach us that most of the workers—perhaps all of them—feel hurt at one stage or another.

The youth possess power, and the worker has no choice but to acknowledge this in his definitions of situations in individual encounters and in the course of his career. The core of their power is their ability to withhold cooperation.

In this chapter we have examined three types of hurt: legitimate non-cooperation (passive avoidance); illegitimate non-cooperation (failure to perform tasks and duties); and disruption (talking without permission during evening meetings).

NOTES

14. On this, see Levy (1993).
15. On "immediacies" in residential child care, see Guttmann (1991).

Chapter 6

The Residential Care Setting
as a Negotiated Order

The situation of the group dictates the course of the residential care
worker's work. When the youth avoid their duties, avoid taking part in
group events or, worse, when they don't listen, when they disrupt or
hurt—the situation tends to disintegrate. In these circumstances the residential care worker has an overwhelming experience of discontent in care: the
world in which he is supposed to fulfill himself professionally is collaps-
ing around him.

This painful experience is something to be avoided, or at least mini-
mized as far as possible. For this to occur, the worker must win his
charges' attention and cooperation; achieving their cooperation becomes
his primary goal. Occupational and personal goals of a higher order, such
as the development and rehabilitation of the youth—not to mention the
worker's own satisfaction and self-actualization—depend on it.

CONTROL

The worker's struggle for the youths' cooperation often takes the form
of various negotiations between them. A typical component of these is
control by the adult residential care worker, the authority figure, over the
youth who are formally subordinate to him. The control process involves
mechanisms for maintenance of consensus on value orientations, or mechanisms that keep motivation at a level and in the direction necessary for

[Haworth co-indexing entry note]: "The Residential Care Setting as a Negotiated Order." Arieli,
Mordecai. Co-published simultaneously in *Child & Youth Services* (The Haworth Press, Inc.) Vol. 18,
No. 2, 1997, pp. 75-93; and: *The Occupational Experience of Residential Child and Youth Care
Workers: Caring and Its Discontents* (Mordecai Arieli) The Haworth Press, Inc., 1997, pp. 75-93. Single
or multiple copies of this article are available for a fee from The Haworth Document Delivery Service
[1-800-342-9678, 9:00 a.m. - 5:00 p.m. (EST). E-mail address: getinfo@haworth.com].

the continuing of the operation of the social system toward its end (Lambert, Millham, & Bullock, 1970, p. 93). In the context of the residential care worker and his tasks, control is the sum of the worker's acts that are designed to make his charges' actions match his goals. Enlisting his charges' participation is, therefore, an act of basic control of them.[16]

Generally, both sides do not seek conflict but wish to maintain a process that will permit them to express to each other their conflicting interests and, with the help of joint interpretive activity, to arrive at a working consensus, or at least a temporary pseudo-concord.[17] In this way the residential setting functions as a negotiated order. And in the framework of the negotiation process, the residential care workers have to try to control their charges. Sometimes they seek control for pedagogic needs, not just for appearances, but sometimes the main purpose is their own survival as residential care workers.

Pedagogic control is designed to serve the interests of the youth—to generate change in them and to help them make effective use of their time. Control for the purpose of survival, on the other hand, serves the interests of the residential care worker: survival in his job means not to be overcome by feelings of discontent, to hold on and not to give up, surrender, or despair because of his charges' actions or inactions.[18]

"Control for survival," despite its importance, is not generally included in the "open pedagogy" taught in training courses. The issue of survival in residential care belongs to the "hidden pedagogy," the residential care workers' informal socialization for their role, which usually occurs after they have started working in that role.

The distinction between the two objectives of control depends on the definitions and interpretations of the workers themselves. Residential care workers may describe their control as pedagogically oriented, while a colleague or a youth observing them will be convinced that the observed interaction was for the purpose of the worker's survival.

In previous chapters, I discussed the residential care workers' perceptions of their work situation, emphasizing their feelings of discontent due to various forms of disruption and hurt, particularly the youths' avoidance of cooperation with them. Now let us look at the workers' attempts to negotiate with their charges to win their cooperation and thus to minimize their own discontent, including the use of various mechanisms of control.

Methods of Control

The ethnographic material reveals seven control methods used by residential care workers in negotiating with the youth to obtain the desired cooperation.[19] The most favored seems to be control by virtue of one's personality, charisma, charm, or by virtue of being considered by the youth to be an epistemic authority, omniscient in the various aspects of their lives as adolescents. Other approaches to controlling include soliciting the youths' interest, building a common middle ground, enlisting the involvement of colleagues, using group management techniques, using organizational authority, and bargaining with the youth to resolve disagreements and move toward shared understandings.

Generally, the residential care worker does not rely on only one control method in a given situation. Some use all seven in their work; others use only one or several of them. Workers were sometimes observed trying three different methods in the course of one ten-minute situation, generally including the last two listed above: the use of authority and bargaining.

All seven approaches are used by residential care workers for additional purposes as well as for control. For example, a worker who is gifted with a charismatic personality may use this advantage to arouse interest and create a middle ground to further his pedagogic beliefs. But here I will quote cases in which these qualities appear to have been used mainly for purposes of control.

Control by Charisma

Charisma appears to be the preferred approach of many residential care workers, who hope–at least at the beginning of their careers–to use this "magical" quality to control their interactions with their charges. The worker hopes that the young people will cooperate with him because of qualities that are not inherent in his work or his actions, but in himself: he fascinates them with his personality and arouses their warm feelings toward him. They like him–and accept his control–because of his amiability, his agreeable manner, his moral qualities, his broad education, his knowledge of the world, his good looks, his youth, his appearance, and/or other qualities that cannot always be acquired and of which they are not always aware or that they cannot define precisely. The youths tend to think of these adult leaders as epistemic authorities on worldly issues and subjects such as politics or sexual conduct.

Thus, the residential care worker hopes that he is worthy of admiration not only for his professional abilities, the interesting activities he organizes, or the benefits to be derived from cooperation with him, and certainly not because of the fear of sanctions to be imposed on one who does not cooperate, but because of who he is.

Benny: We have a new worker, barely 24 years old. We all envy her. Sometimes she makes you feel that working with the kids is the easiest thing in the world for her. It's strange how easily it comes to her. Workers with ten years experience look at her in amazement. They try to learn from her, imitate her, but there doesn't seem to be anything to learn. She doesn't do anything out of the ordinary. I attended one of her group discussions–nothing special.

So what's her secret? It's not a gimmick, it's simply charisma. It's not something she does on purpose. It's more what the kids see in her than anything she does. It's not brains, not warmth, nothing you can pinpoint.

The only rational explanation that somehow comes to mind is that it's connected with what she does outside of her work here and what she plans to do in the future. Most of the residential care workers here are studying for a B.A. in social work, education, psychology, something like that. She's studying business management. She is very happy working here, but she'll almost certainly move on to bigger and better things.

I think the kids here are saying something like: "You want us to take an example from you guys? What for? Maybe one day you'll be senior community workers and you'll have a little apartment somewhere. She's different. She's learning something that will help her to get on in life. She knows what's worth doing. So if we want to be like somebody, it's better to be like her. If anybody here is worth admiring, she's the one!"

Judy: The greatest pleasure in care work is to feel that you are liked just because you're there, that their eyes light up when you smile at them. I'm hooked on that feeling like on a joint, not that I ever touch the stuff . . . I guess I just want to enchant them more than I want to care for them or educate them. There's something very selfish and childish in wanting to be admired by the kids, but I can live with that because I believe that a worker who is admired has a lot of influence and is therefore effective. They envy me because I'm a grasshopper, I try less and succeed more with the kids than the painstaking ants.

But charisma, whatever its source, is not generally a firm basis for cooperation, certainly not an exclusive one. Alongside charisma, most residential care workers find that they have to use other methods of control.

Control by Arousing Interest

The second most preferred basis for gaining control of the youths' cooperation is the ability to arouse their interest. Residential care workers bring to the group meetings various items of equipment designed to serve them as aids. These reflect the residential care worker's didactic approach to the subject he wishes to deal with as well as his way of preparing for a specific meeting.

One such aid is an outline for the meeting, often prepared in the local pedagogic center, a professional resource that operates in many residential care settings in Israel. Preparing such outlines is regarded as professional activity and is often performed as a team assignment guided by more senior residential care workers who specialize in this area. Residential care workers expressed divergent attitudes towards the outline and its preparation. Some thought that:

> *Kedem*: The outline is not realistic. It's almost always over the heads of the kids and sometimes even too complicated for the adults. But you are expected to hold at least some of your group discussions on the basis of it anyway.

> *Dan*: They don't say it in so many words, but in fact they expect the discussion to have learning significance, they expect the kids to learn something new, they expect the residential care workers to act as teachers in a way . . . and all this in the evening, when everyone's tired, when the kids just want to watch a show on TV and relax. No wonder a lot of them don't cooperate. And then they rebel–against whom? Not against those who set the timetable–they're too far away. They rebel against the worker, the one who has to do all that in the evening and often doesn't believe in it any more than they do.

However, other interviewees were convinced of the importance of the activity itself and of preparing for it.

> *Ken*: For the kids who are sent here it's not enough just to give them the same kind of education they would get in regular schools. Their rehabilitation involves building a new world of values, a positive attitude toward the surrounding society, solidarity with society at large. The lessons at school are good for mathematics, English, and computers, not for teaching them values.
>
> If I ask myself why I'm here, one of the main reasons is that I have values and I believe in my ability to transmit them to those who have not received that kind of education in their homes and their natural environment.
>
> The evening meeting is a major tool. Preparing for it ensures that it won't be superficial, boring, or trivial. It's a pity our teachers don't

have a pedagogic center where they can prepare their lessons each day and make sure they won't be boring and mechanical. An educator who comes prepared is a good educator. An educator who is slapdash in a lesson or an activity (and there are some like that here, too, unfortunately) encourages the kids to stagnate rather than change.

Thus, beyond their use as tools to achieve control and cooperation, planning the activity and preparing an outline so as to arouse interest are sometimes presented as didactic acts. Furthermore, they are sometimes perceived as expressions of educational "mission" and "sincerity." The youth are seen as cooperating because the worker is interesting, spontaneous, and frank in private conversations with them and his group activities are well planned, interesting, and successful.

But the residential care worker discovers that when he tries to secure his charges' cooperation, he cannot always rely on his ability to arouse interest, his preparation for the meeting, and his sense of mission. Therefore, he exchanges his hope of gaining their cooperation through charisma or interest for the attempt to achieve it by pleasant or smooth cooptation.

Control by Constructing a Middle Ground

Interviewees described many situations where colleagues adopted parts of their charges' culture to enhance both their negotiating position and their control of the youth so as to win their cooperation. In other words, in order to promote their aims, some residential care workers attempt to appropriate parts of the youth culture by constructing a concrete and symbolic middle ground between their own culture and that of the youth. It is on this culturally unified or shared middle ground that future negotiations between the two groups will take place.[20]

This common cultural territory is perceived by residential care workers as convenient territory from which to persuade their charges gently of the advantages of cooperation, in what appears to be a kind of cooptation. They sometimes develop this middle ground as a first strategy, and sometimes after finding that charisma and/or the interest they are able to arouse are not enough to control their charges. Persuasion based in the middle ground may have various expressions.

Persuasion of the Benefits of Cooperation

Kedem: I heard a residential care worker talking to some of his group in the dining room. They had finished eating and seemed to be just chatting. The same old subject: why should they study and work hard here if their prospects for being able to continue their education after high school are not very good? My colleague spoke to them directly, like one talks to a friend: "So what if you don't continue? You'll get a certificate saying you completed 12 years of schooling. In this country, that's important. The army, for example, won't accept you to any unit worth spending three years of your life on if you haven't graduated. It pays to stick it out here and keep on the good side of everybody–including me–for the sake of finishing twelve years of school. You do it for your own good."

The worker quoted here by his colleague is trying, not in the evening meeting but in the informal situation of a leisurely chat after a meal, to convince his charges that cooperation with him is in their own interest. In these circumstances residential care work will exchange the demand to follow their instructions on "principle" for a request to act according to practical considerations: it's worth listening to what the residential care workers say, not because their authority has to be respected, but because it pays.

Sharing with the Youth. Residential care workers often enlist their charges' cooperation by sharing with them, sincerely or otherwise, certain decisions regarding the running of the group, choosing subjects for evening meetings, and leading that activity. This policy is sometimes guided by progressive values and ideas, based on the belief that the youth's identity will not be rehabilitated by following clear and detailed instructions on what to do every day and every minute of his life but through building an inner base that will give him varied possibilities for autonomous choice of lines of action (Levy, 1993).

However, this important principle sometimes serves the residential care workers not as an objective in itself but as a means of control. Denscombe (1985), discussing the actions of teachers in the classroom, describes this as an act of cooptation. For our purposes, this involves enlisting the youths' willing cooperation–involving them in the running of the group–in the guise of "egalitarian," "liberal," "democratic" attitudes. This kind of sharing, which is not an end in itself but is done for its side benefits, may turn out to be a double-edged sword: a committee elected by the youth may take decisions and use the authority given it by the residential care workers in a way that endangers the workers' control of the group; an individual may exploit the freedom of choice as freedom for anarchy.

Other residential care workers speak of "self-government" either in anger or with cynical remarks. They say that youth councils and committees are declared to be autonomous bodies, expressions of youth culture, but in fact, and as they think the youngsters often feel, these bodies are highly controlled organizational formations.[21]

The youth who tend to join the youth governing bodies are the ones who succeed at school. Some workers claimed that youth join these bodies as a way of rewarding and supporting adults in authority who have "diagnosed" them as good pupils and who have an ideological interest in these "pretenses of democracy." Youth from less advantaged social backgrounds, on the other hand, are rarely "diagnosed" as successful. They tend to reject the adults' expectations. One of the expressions of this is their antagonism toward youth councils and toward accepting "sponsored" roles. One interviewee said rather harshly:

> *Nira*: A kid needs to be a bit of a flatterer for this, a bit of an opportunist. Those who participate in the youth council are the teachers' pets. You won't find many there who don't do well at school.

Role distancing. Another prevalent form of control through cooptation is role distancing, in the sense described by Goffman (1961). This refers to the residential care worker's distancing himself from his formal role as determined by his superiors in the organization, publicly emphasizing his human characteristics in face of the bureaucratic pressures working in the other direction, and adopting symbolic and concrete gestures of approach to the youths' world and culture, perhaps even identifying with them. The worker "enters" the role of the youth, "blending the formal with the informal" (Woods, 1990). Some residential care workers, according to the interviewees, believe that distancing themselves from the role of residential care worker and approaching the role of the youth will help them to be accepted by their charges. Thus, the question sometimes becomes, "Who is coopting whom?"

Interviewees referred to three prevalent expressions of role distancing: imitation, humor and changing the goals of the activity.

Imitation. Residential care workers adopt behaviors that are designed to lend them characteristics similar to those of their charges. Imitation sometimes takes the form of adopting the youth culture's characteristic patterns of discourse. This appears to be common among residential care workers of all ages, not only among the younger ones. Many workers tend to believe that they know the language of the youth culture well enough to adopt it in a way that sounds "natural and spontaneous." Sometimes the imitation takes another form, such as style of dress or hair, and sometimes it consists of trying to join the youth in their informal leisure activities.

Humor. Residential care workers use various forms of joking and humor to get closer to their charges. By making them laugh, the worker hopes to achieve tension-release and to be thought to be friendly and, therefore, to be popular. By making them laugh, they think, they can modify the youths' image of them as custodians.[22]

Changing the goals of the evening meeting. The evening meetings are supposed to serve as stepping-stones toward the achievement of long-term educational objectives. However, many of the meetings are detached from these objectives and designed, in fact, to "pass the time." Many of the activities are more like rituals or games than contributions to the achievement of objectives beyond the interaction actually taking place. Abandoning the original objective of the evening meeting and replacing it with "time-killing" activities in the circumstances of tension or boredom may serve as a role distancing strategy.

Role Distancing as a Double-Edged Sword

Role distancing action such as imitation, joking and replacing the goals of the evening meeting with tension-release activities sometimes succeeds, and the residential care worker gains acceptance and cooperation. But interviewees describe these actions as double-edged swords. Attempts to get closer do not always succeed and sometimes they do exactly the opposite and lead to rejection of the residential care worker.[23]

> *Batya*: One day last week he came into the dining room wearing a T-shirt that was sort of "in" a couple of years ago. You should have heard the whistling and laughter . . . On top of that, he tries to speak in their language, but that doesn't work either. He uses expressions that went out several years ago. It just makes him look ridiculous and they really get off on that.

> *Judy*: You have to admit it. He really is funny and he makes them laugh . . . It helps him a lot at work but sometimes his jokes get on their nerves. A residential care worker is a bit of a father to them, after all . . . It's all right for a father to laugh sometimes . . . , but life is serious, too, so it's frightening to see that your residential care worker-father's major talent is to make you laugh.

> *Jacob*: I can understand situations where the evening meeting fails. It's hard to keep the kids occupied with serious things in the evening. But if that's the situation–fight it. Don't "solve" the problem by turning every activity into a joke. Your kids won't like it.
> I think that's why Sandy failed. He tried to please his group and they

seemed to like it at first. But in the end it turned out that the kids don't respect a worker who bases his activities on ignoring the rules of the place he works in and constantly gives in to the wishes and expectations of his group.

Control Through Involving Colleagues or Sharing with Them

Some of the residential care workers raised the point that a central factor in the residential care worker's "discontent" at work, one that even hinders his ability to control his charges' cooperation, is the fact that in many residential settings he is the lone adult with his group for a whole work shift.

> *Vardi*: It's hard by yourself. You can't make decisions, you can't cope. You need . . . another significant adult, not to share the technical side of the work, but to help you feel less alone in your daily encounters with the kids . . .
> Last year I worked with Gina, an older woman, not the most brilliant in the world, but very warm and experienced. To be honest, she didn't do very much. Most of the time she sat there knitting and listening or dozing. But . . . I learned a lot from her. Sometimes she would look at some of the kids who were acting up. Just one look and they calmed down. On Fridays she used to invite me to her house. Over a cup of coffee she would make a few tactful suggestions. What can I tell you?—she made a residential care worker out of me.

Other interviewees spoke of the advantages of regular support groups to enable workers to share their daily experiences.

> *Hilla*: I try to reach some kind of intimacy with my group. It's hard for me when another adult, even a formal supervisor, takes away part of that intimacy. But I need other adults, especially my colleagues, to share my difficulties after work. At the university they talk a lot about the reflective practitioner, the one who looks at himself and his work and learns from his experience. They say that the reflective practitioner needs other people to maintain what they call reflective interaction. It seems to me that that's what we do here. We meet once or twice a week for two or three hours, not to talk about the kids, but to talk about ourselves in the light of our personal experiences with them. If I'm able to cope with my problems at work, it's because I have people I can talk to about my problems . . . not a supervisor or

some professional wizard but people sharing my daily bread, doing the same job as I am.[24]

Thus, the residential care worker copes with the situation of being a lone adult facing a group of young people by enlisting his colleagues, including those who are not connected with his group, and using them either for consultation or for actual control.

Control by Administrative Preoccupation and Group Management

An alternative approach, used mainly when cooperation is not achieved by charisma, arousing interest, didactic skill, constructing a middle ground, or involving colleagues, is to resort to administrative and group management techniques. The use of group management to achieve cooperation is characterized by a preference for closed interaction, structured, planned, and easy to control, over open interaction that is liable to swing the group unpredictably in any direction.

In various contexts, interviewees voiced the argument that open, free, and spontaneous interaction between the residential care worker and his charges supports developmental and pedagogic goals, but that closed, planned, and administered interaction has the advantage of combatting the technical conditions that permit the youth to avoid cooperation. Patterns of group management designed to help the residential care worker in ensuring cooperation are routinization of the group life and keeping the youth busy most of the time.

Routinization. By this term I mean the tendency of some residential care workers to conduct their interactions with the youth according to a regular and set pattern. This pattern includes a fixed and uniform order and sequence of administrative and educational actions, sometimes with time segments allocated to each.

Adherence to routine seems to make things easier for the worker and frees him of the need to use imagination and invent creative solutions. Regular and fixed activities are conducted like rituals: getting the youths up in the morning, supervision of homework, getting ready for bed. What maintains these rituals is largely the workers' need for regularity and security in a world where they are exposed to unexpected moves from their partners to the interaction.[25]

Keeping Them Busy

Kedem: What is the biggest danger to the routine in the residential setting? I would say idleness. Youngsters who hang around in the afternoon doing nothing, just messing around, kids who don't study, don't work, don't do chores, don't watch TV. They cause trouble for themselves and for the worker. The first time I caught my kids smoking pot and I asked them why the hell they were doing it, they said they were bored.

To some of the residential care workers, "keeping them busy" is a most important organizational-pedagogic principle in the residential setting.[26]

Control Based on Role-Authority

Often, when the five strategies reviewed: charisma, arousing interest, constructing a middle ground, sharing with colleagues, and group management, do not succeed, the residential care worker tries to "discipline" his charges, that is, he tries to use the authority invested in his role to exert control by enforcing rules of behavior. Thus, he imposes his definition of the situation on his charges on the basis of the organizational authority vested in him. Goffman (1961) suggests that staff members in a "total institution" have the authority to impose sanctions with regard to many behavioral items, such as dress, social contact and, in extreme cases, breaking the silence during meals and turning the eyes away during prayers.

Despite the structural similarity of the residential care settings discussed here to total institutions, they are generally very different in their goals and their regime. Mostly, the staff member has no authority, sanction, or administrative need to treat his charges in the ways described by Goffman (1961) in his famous treatise. Most of the disciplinary acts in residential care settings can be described as "deviance imputation" (Hargreaves, Hester, and Mellor, 1975) or implied deviance imputations.

> *Batya*: Generally there's no need to punish. It's enough for me to hint to a kid that he's out of line and he stops what he's doing. It's enough for me to call his name out loud; sometimes it's enough to point to him and then at my lips as a hint for him to be quiet. With me, the expression "read my lips" is not meant as a joke. But I rarely have to punish. I just hint that I want them to behave and the kid will stop talking at once, or get up, or go to bed, or clean his room.

Less common acts of discipline are threats of sanctions; a fairly common threat appears to be the threat to move a youth to another room.

> *Uzzi*: . . . And it almost always works. When I say, "You're not behaving the way you should, I'm moving you to another room,"

what I'm saying is that I'll work against the feeling of home you have found here, I'll remove you from your close little world. This is a cruel threat and it's rarely carried out. But it is one of the most effective acts of discipline we can use. And in very rare cases we actually do it.

Even harsher is the threat to suspend them and send them home, except that this threat is a double-edged sword.

Tal: I never threaten to throw anyone out of the setting. I learned my lesson. I once did threaten a girl and she disappeared. That was exactly what she had been hoping for for months. There are many here who want to go home. They are capable of driving me up the wall so that they'll be sent back to the home they don't really have.

However, in many cases acts of discipline are effective ways of controlling the youths' cooperation. The interviewees mention several reasons for this.

First, the youth in the residential setting identify the place primarily as the territory of the staff. Despite their weaknesses, the staff derive power from their "ownership" of the place, power that enables them to threaten sanctions and impose them.

Hilla: They say to me, "Of course, you're the boss here so you can tell us what to do."

Second, many of the youth come from social groups that are at least ambivalent toward authority figures. On the one hand, these represent social establishments with whom one finds it hard to identify. On the other, one should have respect for adults and for authority figures.

Yehuda: It's rather funny but the fact that we are older than them—sometimes only a little bit older—is more effective than persuasion. So when I shout they shut up.

Batya: Maybe they don't like our demands, but the fact that we seem to have authority has a strong effect. You don't cheek the boss. So when I show that I'm angry and I'm getting ready to punish them they usually try to behave properly.

Sometimes the individual's peers control his behavior toward the person in authority.

Henry: The rule is that you don't just cheek a care worker or any other adult without a good reason. The first to be against someone who does are often the other guys in the group.

Third, according to the interviewees it appears that residential care settings often adopt a certain characteristic of the Goffmanian total institution: unacceptable behavior in one area is liable to affect your status in another area (Goffman, 1961). The youth feel that it is better to respond to the worker's demands for discipline because ignoring them might entail sanctions in another area of life, such as the school.

Tal: Here it's just like Goffman's description. The territorial boundaries between work, sleep, and play disappear. A boy masturbated and left stains on the sheet–and somehow the woman in charge of the library heard about it. How? The em-bayit noticed it and "confided" in her . . .

Tal: Sometimes one of the kids says to me, "O.K., I'll do what you say–just don't tell my teacher." I've also heard colleagues of mine saying to a lad, "Just wait. You won't think you're so clever when they hear about this at school!"

Fourth, the residential care workers naturally receive some backing from the management. The youth are aware of this, just as they are aware that the worker has to try to keep up the appearance that things are under control and therefore it's not wise for him to ask his superiors for backing or intervention too often.

Felix: A girl says to me, "Of course the director will support your decision, but how many times can you go to him for help before he understands that you can't manage on your own?"

Control by Bargaining

And again, the youth–or so residential care workers often hope at the beginning of their careers–will not challenge their right to cooperation if the workers are supported by their colleagues and superiors. Thus, the impression that arises from the interviews is that the residential care workers believe that so long as they exert their authority and act according to the demands of the organization, they are assured of the backing of their colleagues and the director. They know precisely how and in what circumstances to refer a youth who has misbehaved to the administrators.

But there seems to be growing awareness that the authority formally granted them does not solve everything, that the procedures are not always enough, and that they sometimes need to mobilize additional resources. In the fairly early stages of their careers, the workers become aware not only that their personal resources–their talents and skills–do not guarantee their charges' cooperation, but also that resources provided by the organization itself–their status and formal role in the setting and the solidarity of colleagues and superiors–do not guarantee it. Sometimes they find that the power of the youth as individuals, and certainly as a group, is equal if not superior to their power as residential care workers. In that situation, cooperation may be achieved, if at all, only through bargaining for an agreement whereby each side has the ability to influence and moderate the actions of the other.

The youth, too, generally arrive at the same awareness of the necessity for bargaining. A residential care setting is not an organization to which they come completely freely or by chance; it is a framework designed to answer a vital need but it also presents demands. Bargaining differs from negotiating in that it is always direct and somewhat rough or unrefined. Unlike control through constructing a middle ground based on "soft" negotiations or discreet manipulation of the other side, bargaining is an open transaction, give and take. Each side is constantly aware that the other has power and seeks to use it to achieve his objectives and interests in so far as his real and symbolic resources allow him. Both sides aim to reach a consensus, while each tests his strength against the strength of the other.

In regular negotiations each side acts independently of the other side. Even when dialogue is openly conducted they deny its existence. They do not declare an explicit intention to compromise, although each side feels compelled to give up part of his objectives and interests and attempts to exact an adequate return from the other side (Strauss, 1978). In bargaining the dialogue is open. Both sides decrease their original demand on the basis of open recognition of the other side's resources and options.

The residential care workers' demand for cooperation is generally a demand for the youths to adjust and make efforts; the youths' demand to minimize tasks and duties is often a demand for the residential care workers to recognize the legitimacy of components of their lives such as "hanging out," "messing around," and "having fun," however these themes may be operationalized.

The youths recognize the residential care worker's goals, his interest in fulfilling his role, and the personal and organizational resources at his disposal, and they are ready to submit their wishes to his provided that he recognizes their goals and interests and their strength. The residential care worker recognizes his charges' needs and preferences and their reluctance to make efforts and he is prepared to consider them or compromise provided they let him fulfill his role at least ritually, symbolically, and minimally, and show him respect.

> *Kedem*: I said to them, "Look, I hold these pre-army discussions every year and the kids don't find it boring, they don't think it's unimportant. So don't give me that. In six months, most of you will be in the army and you may as well be ready for it . . . All right, I'll keep it light, but don't think you're getting out of it."

> *Asher*: We had an explicit agreement. They could go out in their free time to the nearby town after I had checked that the dorms were clean and tidy. I can't say that they kept their side of the agreement perfectly, but at least they did something and the dorms stopped looking like a pigsty in the afternoon. If they go halfway I'm willing to meet them halfway.

> *Tal*: Then I said, "You want dancing parties? O.K., but let's see you move your butts a little first. Before every party, the whole group goes on three 3-mile hikes at three miles an hour."
> They grumbled, but they agreed. The first hike was a joke. Nobody could do it but me. But I'm trying to be good-hearted, so I kind of gave in to them. Only twice before each party, only two miles, only the boys. And everyone at his own speed. That was the deal. And that was exactly what I wanted in the first place.

In bargaining with youths known to possess considerable power, the residential care worker sometimes prefers to pretend to accept the youth's definition of the situation.

> *Batya*: When you bargain you have to be realistic and know when to give in. I have to ask myself how important the thing really is to me. How far can the kid insist on his demands? It's not worth messing with someone who's very popular over small matters. The price is too high. A residential care worker has to be realistic and sometimes let himself be persuaded or give in.
> About a month ago I "forgot" I had asked a girl who is very popular to stay in the setting on a vacation weekend and look after the group property. She had been out of line for several weeks, and staying in the setting was to be half duty and half punishment . . . but I was

afraid to insist. In the end, I was not quite fair and asked another girl who's easier to deal with.

Was it to the girl's advantage to be relieved of her punishment? Perhaps not. Pedagogues may claim that perhaps it would have been better for this girl to be punished and learn to adjust to the legitimate demands of those in authority. But the residential care worker helped her to avoid it and "work the system." Immunity was given to the more powerful student, the one who might endanger cooperation, but not to the "weaker" one.

Thus, the seventh method used by residential care workers to gain control is bargaining with their charges to resolve disagreements and overcome unpleasant incidents—to avoid, hide or limit them—and replace them with agreements for cooperation. These agreements may be stable and open or, more often, transitory and covert.

> *Jai iih* At first I'm nice to them. If that doesn't work, I try to prove to them that it's worth their while to do what I tell them to. If that doesn't work either, I use discipline—and that usually works.

> *Felix*: Unfortunately, my experience has shown me that you have to give them a short rein. When they behave well, I'm nice to them, but not until then.

> *Asher*: In youth care, being nice is not what it's about. Your authority as a worker doesn't always work. It's better to recognize that they have power and work out some kind of deal with them. Give way to them here and there and they'll give way to you here and there. Then, if you're lucky, you'll be accepted for what you are as well.

The first of the residential care workers quoted here follows the path described above (even if he does not go through every stage): building a shared middle ground with his charges, presenting the instrumental advantages inherent in responding to him, enforcing his authority. The second worker starts by enforcing authority and, if he succeeds, he starts to build a middle ground. The third worker believes in bargaining. If that succeeds, he can then try to use charisma. Control by bargaining does not lead to permanent arrangements, but despite its inherent disadvantages it seems to be an effective way of achieving good "industrial relations" for a while.

CONCLUSION: CONTROL, COOPERATION, AND RULES

In this chapter we have reviewed seven methods used by residential care workers in their endeavors to secure cooperation with their charges:

charisma, arousing interest, constructing a middle ground, involving colleagues, management, discipline, and bargaining. Although charisma is favored, these methods do not form a route that residential care workers follow step by step, from charisma to bargaining. Often they start with attempts at control based on a less favored method.

In six of the seven approaches, the workers make use of their personalities and the talents and skills they have developed. Only one, the sixth, is based mainly on the organization and their official role in it, whereby workers exercise control through authority that the residential care setting gives them.

Residential care workers try to achieve cooperation through rules. The youth are supposed to respond to the workers, who are, therefore, entitled to try to coerce them into participating; the role and place of the youths in the organization forbid deviant behavior and the worker is entitled to demand conformity.

But these rules, it seems, are not clearly and precisely formulated in the regulations of residential care settings. Despite their vagueness, however, the belief in their existence is widespread. It may be that adherence to this belief expressed the workers' need for a feeling of regularity and order in their world. Their belief in the existence of rules regulating life in the residential care setting permits them to describe their course of action to themselves and others as rational and not arbitrary.

Residential care settings, along with many other organizations, have rules whose practical uses seem hard to predict and, in fact, it is not clear in what circumstances they would have practical uses. These are not rules that are likely to shape the actions of those who uphold them, or of those who believe they exist, or of those whose behavior is supposed to be controlled by them. The rules that order the youths' participation in the residential care setting present an even more complex difficulty because of the rarity of precise definitions.

There are some, like Gouldner (1964), who claim that the meaning of the rules is not inherent in their general *a priori* definition, to the extent that this really exists, but in the situation and social context in which somebody sees fit to invoke them. Gouldner sees rules as responses to crises in social relations, a kind of defense against the tensions that arise between people when the expectations of both sides do not match or complement each other.

Rules, according to this approach, are tools for use; when the other available means of supervision and control have been exhausted, they rise to their users' attention, not because they were formulated in advance but in response to the difficulties experienced. Their meaning derives from the definitions of those who invoke them in response to hitches occurring in specific situations and contexts.

It seems, therefore, that when residential care worker-youth interaction proceeds without major snags, some of the youths regularly cooperate with their worker and most respond to his words or acts from time to time. These youth are also permitted to cut off contact with the residential care worker and to do their own thing, living most of the time at a distance from him.

NOTES

16. Hunter (1980) sees the very use of the term "participation" as rhetorical with political and control significance. The word "participation" is designed to encourage youths to be involved in the process known as "their social development" and to encourage educational staff to extend their influence beyond the traditional areas. On the practical level, the term gives legitimization to forms of social control: through it they seek to involve teachers in decisions that were not made by them and to adapt students to socialization in a narrower sense than social development (p. 213).

17. On this interactive process, see Hargreaves (1972).

18. On the meaning of survival at work as the goal of teachers, see Woods (1990).

19. There may, of course, be others to which the interviewees did not refer or which were not identified in the analysis.

20. On teachers' building a middle ground between them and their students, see Woods (1990).

21. See Note 16.

22. On "making them laugh" in the classroom by teachers (and students) and its use as a means of getting closer, enlisting cooperation and control, see, for example, Goodson and Walker (1991), Stebbins (1980), Walker and Gordon (1977), and Woods (1976; 1983).

23. Polsky (1962) describes a case, apparently rare, that marks the danger of approaching through imitation. A residential care worker couple in a care setting wanted to get closer to their wards by adopting some characteristics of their culture. In the course of these endeavors they underwent a process of cooptation by the wards: instead of adjusting the wards to their culture, the care workers adopted characteristics of the delinquent youth culture.

24. This issue is discussed by Fulcher (1991).

25. On the meaning of fixed and uniform order and sequence of controlling actions in the classroom, see Kashti, Arieli, and Harel (1984).

26. On keeping the students constantly occupied as an educational or control strategy in teaching, see Marland (1975) and Millham, Bullock, and Cherrett (1975).

Chapter 7

Care, Contentment, and Commitment

Interviews with residential care workers revealed that, alongside the professional satisfaction they derive from their charges' response, development, and progress, they often derive contentment from their work in two additional ways, rooted in power and human interaction, respectively.

CONTENTMENT IN POWER

Residential care workers reported contentment whose source is the power they have managed to accumulate in their work. They spoke of a state of contentment resulting simultaneously from self-empowerment and empowerment of their charges.

Foucault's analysis regarding power and the formation of social identities can, perhaps, help to illuminate this. Smart (1985:77) suggests that according to Foucault:

> Power is not conceived as a property or possession of a dominant class, state, or sovereign but as a strategy; the effects of domination associated with power arise not from appropriation and deployment by a subject but from "maneuvers, tactics, techniques, functionings"; and a relation of power does not constitute an obligation or prohibition imposed upon the "powerless," rather it invests them, is transmitted by and through them. In short, Foucault conceptualized power neither as an institution nor a structure but as a "complex strategical situation," as a "multiplicity of force relations," as simultaneously "intentional" yet "nonsubjective." The establishment

[Haworth co-indexing entry note]: "Care, Contentment, and Commitment." Arieli, Mordecai. Co-published simultaneously in *Child & Youth Services* (The Haworth Press, Inc.) Vol. 18, No. 2, 1997, pp. 95-106; and: *The Occupational Experience of Residential Child and Youth Care Workers: Caring and Its Discontents* (Mordecai Arieli) The Haworth Press, Inc., 1997, pp. 95-106. Single or multiple copies of this article are available for a fee from The Haworth Document Delivery Service [1-800-342-9678, 9:00 a.m. - 5:00 p.m. (EST). E-mail address: getinfo@haworth.com].

95

and implementation of such relations of power is directly correlated with the production and circulation of true discourse.

Following Foucault, the residential care worker, like everybody in every human situation, does not receive the power of his role as a property or possession and cannot take it for granted. He has to attain it through "maneuvers, tactics, techniques, functionings."

The sense of power tends to influence the residential care worker's previous definitions of the situation and, with them, the strategies he employed in his interactions with his charges. The residential care worker who experiences power is likely from now on to discover that he is less vulnerable and that many behaviors he hitherto defined as hurts or disruptions are expected responses of partners in human interactions. From now on, he will conclude or feel that, although these actions are guided by personal or collective interests (like most human actions in any collective context), they are not necessarily intended to hinder or prevent cooperation. In these circumstances the residential care worker may dare to replace the orientation that guides his interactions with his charges from control based on "power over" the youth to a symmetrical dialogue based on "power with" the youth.

The distinction between "power over" and "power with" in adult-youth relations in educational contexts was suggested by Kreisenberg (as mentioned in Bloome & Willett, 1991). "Power over" is power in the usual sense of the word: one side has power which it uses to restrict the other side. In contrast, in "power with" relations, empowered educators make use of their authority and competence to empower their students to realize their rights and competence.

TO BE WITH PEOPLE

Usually the stated objective of the encounter between residential care workers and their charges is the education and care of the youths. They—and consequently, society at large—are the main intended beneficiaries of the anticipated results of the encounter. But some of the workers mentioned an additional angle, an aspect that yields contentment not directly connected with the benefits for the young people and for society: contentment from the close contact with people—particularly the youth—that the residential care situation provides abundantly.

Their confrontations with their charges provide the workers with numerous opportunities to talk with others about almost every subject that concerns them, such as cultural, social, and political issues and, often indirectly, about existential questions with which they are engaged. It is not only the evening meetings that provide them with an audience and partners for discussion, but every casual encounter may serve as a context for exploration and self-questioning. Working with the youth is an opportunity to be with people and to share your world with them.

COPING WITH DISCONTENT

The previous chapter enumerated seven ways used by residential care workers to deal with youths who cause them discontent or to control their actions. In addition to their direct confrontation with the youths, the workers develop reflective coping methods—ways of coping that do not limit the youths as partners to the interaction to decrease their discontent. In these coping methods the individual residential care worker is simultaneously both the subject (the one doing the thinking) and the object of his considerations (the one he is thinking about).

Two mechanisms that appear to be the most prevalent, "everyday" ones for reducing discontent by reflective methods are: (1) replacing the primary commitment to one's work with secondary commitment; and (2) imputing youths' acting out against them to transference, that is, development of a belief that disruption, hurtful, and similar behaviors of the youth are often acts that are not really directed against the worker but against the parental figure whom he represents or symbolizes in the depths of their being.

From Primary to Secondary Commitment

Although I believe that every microsocial event can be explained, at least partly, by the circumstances of the macrosocial context, the residential care workers' shift from primary to secondary commitment appears to require particular clarification in terms of the circumstances of its social context. Therefore, the present discussion of this process will be prefaced by a few lines on the macrosocial context of residential care workers in Israel including, of course, those who were interviewed for this study. More broadly, I believe that the process has significance beyond the boundaries of the Israeli culture, as will be explained below.

In Jewish society in Palestine during the British Mandate (1922-1948) and in the early years after the State of Israel was established in 1948, most of the residential educational settings in Israel were designed to generate change in their charges; they were "people-changing" more than "people-processing" organizations (Arieli, Kashti, & Shlasky, 1983). A similar objective was, and at least officially still is, the policy of most residential settings in Europe and North America.

The "powerful environment" of the Israeli residential educational setting sought to resocialize its charges, to mold immigrant youths as Israelis, to change the predicted career of urban Jewish youths from Europe into a future of life on the land, and to bring the youth from North Africa and the Middle East into the mainstream culture of the nascent Israeli society with its western orientation. Therefore, the youths were exposed to pressure to exchange their accustomed patterns of education and culture, in whose spirit they had been socialized, for new patterns derived from the pioneering, Zionist, and mostly socialist ethos.

Residential educational settings in Israel often trained their pupils to be part of a social *avant-garde*. From this point of view, the histories of the kibbutz movement and of the Jewish defense organizations are linked with the histories of agricultural schools, youth villages, and kibbutz youth groups.

Their resocialization in the residential settings brought the youth to take up important social roles. These roles were undertaken, in the nature of things, quite autonomously, but clearly the youth were exposed both to the pressure of the setting and to hidden pressure from their peers to conform to the ethos of pioneering and defense. The impression received is that informal sanctions were often imposed on "deviants" from this ethos.

After the establishment of the State of Israel in 1948 and particularly in recent decades, many residential educational settings have become places for the advancement and rehabilitation of the so-called "socially disadvantaged" or "culturally deprived" youth. Thus, at least ostensibly, the residential educational setting continues to act as a resocialization agent for its wards, but youth from established socioeconomic backgrounds, particularly in the non-religious sector, often eschew residential education—and certainly care—and thus avoid social integration with residential pupils in after-school hours even when they go to school together.

In addition, the percentage of residential pupils, compared with regular day school students, who pass the matriculation exams, which are a necessary precondition for academic higher education in Israel, is usually rather low. These two facts cast doubt on the continued ability of residential settings to resocialize their wards and to promote their upward social mobility. Moreover, it may be that residential care and education settings act unintentionally to stabilize and perpetuate their residents' status (compared with their parents) and, thus, that they function as organizations of social reproduction.[27]

The gradual transition of many Israeli residential schools from resocializing organizations to settings that stress care rather than schooling has affected the role and status of the worker in the residential setting. Henceforth he is not the ideological representative of a movement, a central agent of the host society in the process of cultural transition to a new society, and an attractive figure for imitation and identification. His role now focuses on performing diffuse tasks of organizational coordinator, custodian, teacher's aide helping the younger children with their homework. Although he was never a professional in the conventional sense of the word, some of the developmental aspects of his role are now replaced by custodial elements, and group leadership is often superseded by focusing on the needs of the individual youth. The change in the residential care worker's role is reflected in a gradual change in his status from being a disseminator and agent of the ideas of change on behalf of an elite *avant-garde* to being a semi-professional educational worker.[28]

The change in the residential care worker's role and the concomitant change in his status appears to be accompanied by a change in the nature of his commitment to his educational career. In the early days of residential education in Israel, the residential care worker's commitment to his role was characterized by a voluntary approach. "Commitment" to his work did not mean devotion to a regular job but an intensive endeavor to realize social ideals. The worker was often a person with a vocation rather than a bureaucratic performer of routine tasks.

Thus, "commitment" was perceived as the willingness of an individual or a group, for our purposes the residential care workers in educational settings, to devote their energy and loyalty to the interests of the wards of the setting as if they were their own interests. A "committed" person was one who identified the interests of the system for which he acted with his own.[29]

The committed residential care worker deployed his reserves to achieve the objectives of the system and related to them as if they were his own personal goals, or those of the political collective (kibbutz, youth movement) to which he belonged. He did his work with deep conviction of its importance or of the rightness of his educational goals; his approach was usually idealistic and somewhat altruistic. This kind of commitment will be referred to here as primary commitment.

With the change in his role from being an agent of resocialization to being a "care agent," and the accompanying change in his status, the residential care worker exchanged his primary commitment for a commitment whose basis was not free of personal interests. I refer to a situation whereby the worker is primarily committed to his craft because he does not want to waste the investments and the "side bets" (Becker, 1960) that he has made so far in acquiring his occupation and accumulating experience and status in it and in the setting where he works. This kind of commitment I call secondary commitment.[30]

Woods (1989), in discussing survival and nonsurvival in teaching, expresses concern not for those who survive in teaching nor for those who drop out of the profession, but for those in the middle, those who are committed. It seems to me that the commitment he refers to is what I describe as secondary commitment. These are the educational workers who are trapped between loyalty to their work and the pressures of their work. They do not solve their problems as residential care workers by minimizing contact with their charges or leaving the scene of conflict, they do not "compromise" or replace the planned schedule with things that will placate their charges or entertain them. These have nothing left to give, says Woods (discussing teachers) but themselves (Woods, ibid. p. 93).

Like primary commitment, secondary commitment involves the continual deployment of personal resources for the system in which the individual acts and with whose goals he identifies, but it is not totally altruistic or idealistic.

> *Kalia*: I've been in this business for many years. I am experienced. I have no illusions. We have a staff apartment, and my husband has a very senior position here. It would not be easy for us to leave.
>
> But the main thing is, I still believe in these kids and in what I have to give them. A quarter of the time I devote to my work is not effective at all. But in the other three quarters, I give them something that's hard to describe, but I know it's important to them.
>
> I don't expect to be very popular, and I'm not as enthusiastic as I used to be. My faith in these kids' morals and in their chances of improving has its limits, but I'm not completely pessimistic. Nor do I have much of an alternative. So I stay.

Paradoxically, on the face of it the feeling of having no way out becomes a resource. Leaving the residential educational setting or reducing their work activities to the minimum necessary for survival appear to be less attractive choices.

Those with secondary commitment profit by remaining in the organization and lose by leaving it. Their continued work involves "investment" or "sacrifice." The residential care workers have to give up something in order to stay in their jobs and their place of work. This in itself strengthens their commitment. It is hard to give up something in which you have invested and for which you have made sacrifices.

Furthermore, the residential care worker finds himself in a situation of cognitive dissonance in the sense described by Festinger (1957). On the one hand, he experiences frustration and he thinks of abandoning the career of residential care worker; on the other, he does not want to lose what he has already invested in the occupation. To resolve the conflict, he changes his attitude with regard to the frustration. He channels his future actions along courses set out for him by his employers or superiors in the residential educational setting. Thus, he not only distances himself more and more from alternative career options, but he searches for sources of contentment in his job and workplace.

However, the daily lives of residential care workers rob them of their illusions. This is a process the interviewers described as "inevitable." When this happens, the feeling of commitment is replaced by another feeling, that of withdrawal. Workers often said that they now occasionally limit their work to activities designed to "pass the time," to somehow let them get through the day in peace and quiet.

The understanding that progressive ideals do not always match reality in the residential educational settings led residential care workers to give up their ideals. But this is distressful: it is not a question of giving up a material ambition to attain something outside oneself; it is giving up something that was—at least initially—a significant part of their being. Those who hold educational conceptions and try to act accordingly are often called "idealists," meaning people for whom material reward is of secondary value, people who are prepared to devote themselves whole-heartedly to goals that do not directly serve their interests. For these people, giving up their ideals means giving up an important part of their "selves."

Perhaps the residential care workers' relinquishing of their ideals as a result of discovering the nature of reality is like such discovery in any other aspect: life is not as glorious as the dream. But apparently in the case of the residential care workers, it is aggravated by the fact that they constantly make this discovery anew in interactions whose dynamics follow a pattern for which it is impossible to prepare and that is impossible to avoid.

It's Not Me; It's the Person Whose Role I Play in the Youth's Life

Selected ideas from psychodynamic literature that are considered relevant are presented to residential care workers explicitly or implicitly in training and refresher courses conducted in various countries—particularly, it seems, in Israel. This psychoanalytic ethos guided generations of residential social pedagogy in the Israeli kibbutz. An idea that apparently acquired a special position in the residential care workers' awareness as a result is the idea of transference.

The theory of transference is based on the observed tendency of individuals to repeat in new relationships patterns set in previous ones. For example, in relationships with a therapist, one tends to repeat patterns set with one's parents at the stage of development that Freud called Oedipal. And thus, say some who are involved in the training of residential care workers, the youth tend to repeat in relationships with residential care workers patterns that were set with their parents at that stage.

According to this approach, the young people's frequent discourse with their residential care workers on intimate subjects recalls earlier intimate experiences. Thus, the worker becomes a parent in the youth's mental imagery. The process is aided by the youth's dependence and his wish to transfer responsibility, knowledge, and control from himself to the worker. Transference can be expressed by falling in love with a worker, usually one of the opposite sex, or by a different highly charged emotional response to everything the worker says or does.

Actually, the youth has little choice but to model his relations with his residential care worker on patterns familiar to him from elsewhere—his home, his neighborhood, etc.; these are all he knows. The transference involves a paradox: on the one hand, its strength is what gives the residential care worker his power; the youth, as it were, asks for parental patronage that will give meaning to his life. Yet on the other hand, the aim of the worker should be to moderate the transference and show that the right place for the emotions involved lies somewhere else altogether, in the youth's relations with his natural parents, in the service of his development. To redirect the relationship in this direction may be difficult for the worker, who can easily be "seduced" by the power and the relationship factors in the situation to reinforce rather than redirect the transference. (In the psychodynamic vernacular, this is often described as "countertransference.")

In any case, during the process the youth's hostility, disruptions, and hurt, and the discontent he causes do not reflect his "accounts" only with the residential care worker, but also with the parental figure or figures whom the worker represents or symbolizes. The worker who is aware of these processes and their meaning will, presumably, feel less discontent in his relations with his charges.

CONCLUSION

The situations described in this volume repeatedly confirm the validity of the approach that guided me: interactions are a central aspect in explaining events in residential settings. Such settings are frameworks in which skilled adults with authority coexist with young people who are seen as needing to be changed and who have little authority. This is the basis of the interactions that occur and it is this that determines the nature of the experience. As I have tried to show, the experience contains many elements of discontent for residential care workers, but elements of contentment emerge together with them or in their wake.

Residential care workers' perspectives regarding their situations and those of their charges and their groups, as they emerge from relevant literature throughout the world (some of which is cited here), are often compatible with the conclusions of researchers who have examined these subjects with tools other than ethnographic interviews. In this sense the descriptions here indirectly confirm, from a different angle, what is known about the situation of the residential care worker in the context of his work. I have focused on how residential care workers experience discontent and may try to minimize or stifle it by employing various strategies to control the youths' definition of the situation and their behavior.

Is it possible to act in such a way as to limit in advance or even prevent the experience of discontent? Or is discontent inherent in care work, accompanying it as an ongoing, immanent experience? These questions were not raised directly by the interviewers but by many of the residential care workers, who see worker discontent as a problem (at least for their colleagues) and wondered about its inevitability and possible solutions.

Toward Enhanced Worker Contentment

Do the interviews provide evidence to support the assumption and hope that there is the possibility of carework without discontent? Some of the workers expressed the opinion that appropriate preparation in three domains may reduce or entirely prevent most of the experiences of discontent in care: reorganization of the residential setting; improvement of carework methods; and special emphasis in the training of residential care workers' on the subject of their interactions with the youth, particularly during practical training (fieldwork). Thus, discontent is not perceived by most of the interviewees as an intrinsic experience that inevitably accompanies a career of care.

Reorganization of the Setting. As regards the first domain, reorganization of the residential setting, the materials and data that serve the present discussion do not shed much light on the residential care workers' assumption concerning the potential contribution of changes in the complex organization of the residential setting to the improvement of relations between residential care workers and their charges. One should be aware of the danger of "macro-blindness," that is, the failure to give sufficient consideration to the part played by organizational circumstances beyond a given situation described, which may interfere with a researcher's perception of the micro-social reality.

Most of the issues mentioned by the residential care workers in the interviews did not, to the best of my knowledge, relate directly or explicitly to the organization of a specific residential setting, no matter what its type, size, or the nature of its residents. A pattern of events described by a residential care worker in one residential setting was often reported by another one in another residential setting with an entirely different organizational size and culture.

Improved Methods of Carework. As for the second domain, the improvement of carework methods, many interviewees stated in different ways that interesting, effective, and meaningful carework is the best remedy to prevent discontent in care. In particular, some of them criticized the evening meeting, saying that it is the formal imposition of an obligation disguised as an informal and even voluntary activity. Some reported effective personal experiences in improving care by developing the residential care worker's professionalism through reflective action: observing himself in action, reflecting on it, and sharing his experiences with colleagues (in workshops, for example).

They consider that these may help to improve their work methods and thus lead to more pleasurable interaction between the residential care workers and their charges. However, other interviewees said that in their experience, good care work is a necessary but not a sufficient condition for positive interaction with their charges and for the residential care workers' contentment.

Training. With regard to the third domain, training for effective interaction with the youth in the general framework of residential care worker training, many of the interviewees saw a link between training for carework and the levels of contentment and discontent. In their opinion, these have their source largely in the methods of formal and informal socialization for the role of residential care worker, and discontent can be prevented or lessened and contentment enhanced by effecting changes in residential care worker training.

CAN THE FINDINGS BE GENERALIZED?

It is not my impression that the overall picture that has emerged from the study reflects a situation that is unique to Israel, or an Israeli residential setting culture that is significantly different from the cultures of other residential settings described in the past twenty years or so in the relevant professional literature in North America and Britain.[31] Thus, it may be possible to state at least tentatively that the findings of this study reflect the reality of residential settings in most modern countries. In other words, perhaps the forces and phenomena that have been documented here extend beyond the specific reality of any one culture.

THE RESIDENTIAL CARE WORKERS' PERSPECTIVE

The examination of the residential care workers' perceptions and understandings of the situations they encounter in their group, and of how they cope with the experience of discontent inherent in many of these situations, required a discussion of a holistic nature. To facilitate this, I tried to put myself in the place of the residential care workers and to discuss their experiences and understandings from their perspective. Thus, I sought to bring the reader into the residential care setting, a world with a rich, variegated, and constantly changing mosaic of interactions. Just as the residential care worker did not focus on selected "variables" in reflecting on the operation of his group and his situation in it, I, too, sought to document his world, if not in its entirety, then at least in many aspects of it.

The residential setting, it appears, is not only a place for development, rehabilitation and education but, like most human frameworks that bring people together, also an arena of power struggles, triumphs and losses, contentment and discontent. Thus, contentment is not necessarily perceived as the opposite of discontent. The opposite of discontent is often merely the absence of discontent, a situation that does not necessarily bring contentment.

Many residential care workers I have spoken to over the years insisted that their own work lives were not problematic or painful, although those of many of their colleagues were; from what they said, one might have concluded that they had barely experienced any real discontent. But even those interviewees who reported personal discontent often stated that they also had ongoing experiences of contentment. Contentment and discontent, it appears, are not mutually exclusive. Residential care settings provide their workers with both types of experience, sometimes simultaneously.

NOTES

27. For a comparison of these processes in the USA and Israel, see Arieli, Kashti, Shapira, Cookson, and Hodges Persell (1988/9).

28. On the processes of change in Israeli residential settings and in the role and status of the residential care worker, see Kashti (1979) and Shlasky (1985).

29. Commitment in general and commitment in education in particular has been extensively discussed in the literature. The discussion of the meaning of commitment in this book largely follows the approaches of Becker (1960, 1964), Freeman (1989), Nias (1981), Sikes, Measor, and Woods (1985), and Woods (1981).

30. Sikes, Measor, and Woods (1985) make a similar distinction, in the educational context, between three commitments: commitment to education as a vocation, professional commitment (to the subject they teach, to teaching as a profession, or to the school) and instrumental commitment (to a career and its practical benefits for the teacher). They suggest that the teachers' commitment tends to change over the years from vocational to professional and from professional to instrumental.

31. A review of this literature can be found in Bullock, Little and Millham (1993).

References

Adler, H., & Shapira, R. (Eds.). (1981). *Residential education in Israel: Report of the Israel-American Seminar on Out-of-School Education.* US-Israel Memorandum of Understanding in Education (item K), 103-110.

Anglin, J.P. (1991). Residential care for children and youth in Canada. In M. Gottesmann (Ed.), *Residential care: An international reader.* London: Whiting & Birch.

Arieli, M. (1989). Students' supportive attitude toward their schools: The case of the youth village and its student society. In E. Krausz (Ed.), *Education in a comparative context. Studies in Israeli society, Vol. IV.* New Brunswick: Transaction.

Arieli, M. (1995). *Teaching and its discontents.* Tel Aviv: Ramot (in Hebrew).

Arieli, M., Kashti, Y., Shapira, R., Cookson, P. W., & Hodges Persell, C. (1988/9). Residential schooling in the US and Israel: the integrative and allocative functions. *Israel Social Science Research, 6*(1), 1-8.

Arieli, M., Kashti, Y., & Shlasky, S. (1983). *Living at school: Israeli residential schools as people processing organizations.* Tel Aviv: Ramot.

Ball, S.J. (1980). Initial encounters in the classroom and the process of establishment. In P. Woods (Ed.), *Pupil strategies: Explorations in the sociology of the school.* London: Croom Helm.

Ball, S.J. (1987). *The micro-politics of the school: Toward a theory of school organization.* London: Methuen.

Becker, H.S. (1960). Notes on the concept of commitment. *American Journal of Sociology, 66,* 32-40.

Becker, H.S. (1964). Personal change in adult life. *Sociometry, 27*(1), 40-53.

Beker, J. (1981). New roles for group care centers. In F. Ainsworth & L.C. Fulcher (Eds.), *Group care for children: Concept and issues.* London: Tavistock.

Beker, J., & Feuerstein, R. (1991). Toward a common denominator in effective group care programming: The concept of the modifying environment. *Journal of Child and Youth Care Work, 7,* 20-34.

Beker, J., & Magnuson, D. (1996). Residential education as an option for at-risk youth: Learning from the Israeli experience. *Residential Treatment for Children and Youth, 13*(3), 3-48. (Also published as J. Beker &

D. Magnuson (Eds.), *Residential education as an option for at-risk youth.* New York: The Haworth Press, Inc., 1996.)

Beynon, J. (1984). Sussing out teachers: Pupils as data gatherers. In M. Hammersley & P. Woods (Eds.), *Life in school.* Milton Keynes: Open University Press.

Beynon, J. (1985). *Initial encounters in the secondary school.* Lewes: Falmer.

Blase, J. (Ed.). (1991). *The politics of life in schools: Power, conflict, and cooperation.* Newbury Park: Sage.

Bloome, D., & Willett, J. (1991). Towards a micropolitics of classroom interaction. In J. Blase (Ed.), *The politics of life in schools: Power, conflict, and cooperation.* Newbury Park: Sage.

Buber, M. (1958). *I and thou.* New York: Charles Scribner's Sons.

Bullock, R. (1993). Child care in the EC: The United Kingdom. In M.J. Colton & W. Hellinckx (Eds.), *Child care in the EC: A country-specific guide to foster and residential care.* Aldershot: Arena, Ashgate.

Bullock, R., Little, M., & Millham, S. (1993). *Residential care for children: A review of the literature.* London: HMSO.

Carlebach, J. (1982). The world of the staff members. *Youth Aliyah Bulletin,* March, 32-42.

Central Bureau of Statistics, Government of Israel (1996). *Boarding schools in post-primary educational institutions, 1991\1992.* Series of Education and Culture Statistics, 212.

Cole, M., & Walker, S. (Eds.). (1989). *Teaching and stress.* Milton Keynes: Open University Press.

Colla-Müller, H. (1993). Child care in the EC: Germany. In: M.J. Colton & W. Hellinckx (Eds.), *Child care in the EC: A country-specific guide to foster and residential care.* Aldershot: Arena, Ashgate.

Collins, R. (1979). *The credential society.* New York: Academic Press.

Colton, M.J., & Hellinckx, W. (Eds.). (1993). *Child care in the EC: A country-specific guide to foster and residential care.* Aldershot: Arena, Ashgate.

Comstock, D. (1982). Power in organizations: toward a critical theory. *Pacific Sociological Review, 25*(2), 139-162.

Davies Jones, H. (Ed., English edition). (1985). *The Social Pedagogue in Europe: Living with Others as a Profession.* Zurich: FICE (Federation Internationale des Communautes Educatives).

Denscombe, M. (1985). *Classroom control: A sociological perspective.* London: George Allen Unwin.

Eisikovits, R.A. (1991). The child care worker as ethnographer: Uses of the anthropological approach in residential child and youth care education and practice. In J. Beker & Z. Eisikovits (Eds.), *Knowledge utiliza-*

tion in residential child and youth care practice. Washington, D.C.: Child Welfare League of America.

Eisikovits, Z. (1986). Changing career patterns in Israeli child care work. *Child & Youth Services, 7*(3/4), 143-156.

Festinger, L. (1957). *A theory of cognitive dissonance.* Evanston, IL: Row-Peterson.

Feuerstein, R. (1987). A foster home and group care experiment. In Y. Kashti & M. Arieli (Eds.), *Residential settings and the community: Congruence and conflict.* London: Freund.

Federation Internationale des Communautes Educatives (FICE). (1990). Survey: Training institutions for child and youth care workers. *FICE International Bulletin* (Autumn).

Freeman, A (1989). Coping and SEN. Challenging idealism In M. Cole & J. Walker (Eds.), *Teaching and stress.* Milton Keynes: Open University Press.

Freud, S. (1930). *Civilization and its discontents.* Standard Edition, Vol. 21.

Frommann, A., Haag, G., & Trede, W. (1991). Residential education in the Federal Republic of Germany. In M. Gottesmann (Ed.), *Residential care: An international reader.* London: Whiting & Birch.

Fulcher, L.C. (1991). Teamwork in residential care. In J. Beker & Z. Eisikovits (Eds.), *Knowledge utilization in residential child and youth care practice.* Washington, DC: Child Welfare League of America.

Furlong, V.J. (1976). Interaction sets in the classroom. In M. Hammersley & P. Woods (Eds.), *The process of schooling.* London: Routledge & Kegan Paul.

Geerts, C. (1975). *The interpretation of culture.* London: Hutchinson.

Goffman, E. (1961). *Asylums.* Hammondsworth: Penguin.

Goldman, R., & Manburg, A. (1985). Relationships among child care professionals: A model of collaborative supervision. *Journal of Child Care, 2(4),* 53-60.

Goodson, I., & Walker, B. (1991). Humour in the classroom. In I. Goodson & B. Walker (Eds.), *Biography, identity, and schooling.* London: Falmer.

Gottesmann, M. (1991a). Professionalization of the residential youth care worker. *FICE International Bulletin* (Federation Internationale des Communautes Educatives), *4,* 48-53.

Gottesmann, M. (Ed.). (1991b). *Residential care: An international reader.* London: Whiting & Birch.

Gottesmann, M. (Ed.). (1994). *Recent changes and new trends in extrafa-*

milial child care: An international perspective. London: Whiting & Birch.

Gouldner, A.W. (1964). About the functions of bureaucratic rules. In A.W. Gouldner, *Patterns of industrial bureaucracy.* New York: The Free Press.

Gouldner, A.W. (1970). "Cosmopolitans and locals": Toward an analysis of latent social roles. In D. Gursky & G.A. Miller (Eds.), *The sociology of organizations: Basic studies.* New York: Free Press.

Guttmann, E. (1991). Immediacy in residential child and youth care: The fusion of experience, self-consciousness, and action. In J. Beker & Z. Eisikovits (Eds.), *Knowledge Utilization in Residential Child and Youth Care Practice.* Washington, DC: Child Welfare League of America.

Hammersley, M., & Turner, G. (1980). Conformist pupils? In P. Woods (Ed.), *Pupil strategies: Explorations in the sociology of the school.* London: Croom Helm.

Hargreaves, D.H. (1972). *Interpersonal relations and education.* London: Routledge & Kegan Paul.

Hargreaves, D.H., Hester, S.K., & Mellor, F.J. (1975). *Deviance in classrooms.* London: Routledge & Kegan Paul.

Hunter, C. (1980). The politics of participation–With specific reference to teacher-pupil relationships. In P. Woods (Ed.), *Teacher strategies: Explorations in the sociology of the school.* London: Croom Helm.

Jackson, P.W. (1968). *Life in classrooms.* New York: Holt, Rinehart and Winston.

Kahan, B. (1994). Review of recent trends in residential and extrafamilial care of children and young people. In M. Gottesmann (Ed.), *Recent changes and new trends in extrafamilial child care: An international perspective.* London: Whiting & Birch.

Kashti, Y. (1979). The socializing community. Tel Aviv: SEE–Studies in Educational Evaluation.

Kashti, Y. (1988). Boarding school and changes in society and culture. *Comparative Education, 24*(3), 351-364.

Kashti, Y. (1991). Residential education and care: A sociological perspective. In M. Gottesmann (Ed.), *Residential care: An international reader.* London: Whiting & Birch.

Kashti, Y., Arieli, M., & Harel, Y. (1984). Classroom seating as a definition of situation. *Urban Education, 19*(2), 161-181.

Keddie, N. (1971). Classroom knowledge. In M.F.D. Young (Ed.), *Knowledge and control.* London: Collier-Macmillan.

Kelly, C. K. (1990). Professionalizing child and youth care: An overview. *Child & Youth Services, 13*(1), 167-177.

Kyriacou, C. (1989). The nature and prevalence of teacher stress. In M. Cole & S. Walker (Eds.), *Teaching and stress.* Milton Keynes: Open University Press.

Lacey, C. (1970). *Hightown grammar.* Manchester: Manchester University Press.

Lacey, C. (1975). *The socialization of teachers.* London: Methuen.

Lambert, R., Bullock, R., & Millham, S. (1973). The informal social system. In R. Brown (Ed.), *Knowledge, education, and culture.* London: Tavistock.

Lambert, R., Millham, S., & Bullock, R. (1970). *Manual to the sociology of the school.* London: Weidenfeld & Nicolson.

Lane, D. (1994). The community and the residential home. In M. Gottesmann (Ed.), *Recent changes and new trends in extrafamilial child care: An international perspective.* London: Whiting & Birch.

Lemert, E.M. (1967). *Human deviance: Social problems and social control.* Englewood Cliffs, NJ: Prentice-Hall.

Levy, Z. (1993). *Negotiating positive identity in a group care community: Reclaiming uprooted youth.* New York: The Haworth Press, Inc. (Also published as *Child & Youth Services, 16*(2), 1993.)

Little, M. (with Kelly, S.). (1995). *A life without problems?* Aldershot, Hants: Ashgate.

Malen, B. (1994). The micro-politics of education: Mapping the multiple dimensions of power relations in school politics. *Politics of Education Association Yearbook, 1994, 147-167.*

Marland, M. (1975). *The craft of the classroom.* London: Heinemann.

Meyer, J.W., Scott, W.R., & Deal, T.E. (1983). Institutional and technical sources of organizational structure: Explaining the structure of educational settings. In J.W. Meyer & W.R. Scott (Eds.), *Organizational environments: Ritual and rationality.* Beverly Hills: Sage.

Millham, S., Bullock, R., & Cherrett, P. (1975). *After grace—Teeth.* London: Human Context, Chaucer.

Nias, J. (1981). Commitment and motivation in primary school teachers. *Educational Review, 33*(3), 181-190.

Pfeffer, J. (1989). *Power in organizations.* Marshfield, MA: Pitman.

Philipson. N. (1972). Phenomenological philosophy and sociology. In P. Filmer et al., *New directions in sociological theory* (pp. 119-165). London: Collier-Macmillan.

Pollard, A. (1985). *The social world of the primary school.* London: Holt, Rinehart & Winston.

Polsky, H. (1962). *Cottage six.* New York: Russell-Sage Foundation.

Powell, D.R. (1990). Professionalism and the child care field. *Child & Youth Services, 13*(1), 177-186.

Raviv, A., Bar-Tal, D., & Peleg, D. (1990). Perception of epistemic authorities by children and adolescents. *Journal of Youth and Adolescence, 19,* 495-510.

Reddin, W.J. (1970). *Managerial effectiveness.* New York: McGraw Hill.

Reynolds, D. (1976). The delinquent school. In M. Hammersley & P. Woods (Eds.), *The process of schooling.* London: Routledge & Kegan Paul.

Sarup, M. (1978). *Marxism and education.* London: Routledge and Kegan Paul.

Schutz, A. (1970). *Reflections on the problem of relevance.* New Haven: Yale University Press.

Searle, J. (1984). *Minds, brains, and science: The 1984 Reith Lectures.* London: Penguin.

Shalom, H. (1980). The role perception of the "madrich" in residential settings. In S. Adiel, H. Shalom & M. Arieli (Eds.), *Fostering deprived youth and residential education.* Tel-Aviv: Gomeh (in Hebrew).

Shapira, R. (1987). Residential settings and the community: Exchange relations. In Y. Kashti & M. Arieli (Eds.), *Residential settings and the community: Congruence and conflict.* London: Freund.

Shlasky, S. (1985). *Occupational choice and career orientations of residential care workers in Israel.* Unpublished Ph.D. Dissertation, Sussex University, UK.

Sikes, P., Measor, L., & Woods, P. (1985). *Teacher careers: Crises and continuities.* Lewes: Falmer.

Silverman, D. (1970). *The theory of organizations.* London: Heinemann.

Smart, B. (1985). *Michel Foucault.* London & New York: Tavistock Publications.

Stebbins, R.A. (1977). The meaning of academic performance: How teachers define a classroom situation. In P. Woods & M. Hammersley (Eds.), *School experience: Explorations in the sociology of education.* London: Croom Helm.

Stebbins, R.A. (1980). The role of humor in teaching: Strategy and self-expression. In P. Woods (Ed.), *Teacher strategies: Explorations in the sociology of the school.* London: Croom Helm.

Stebbins, R. (1981). Classroom ethnography and the definition of the situation. In L. Barton & S. Walker (Eds.), *Schools, teachers, and teaching.* Lewes: Falmer.

Strauss, A. (1978). *Negotiations.* San Francisco: Jossey-Bass.

Tattum, D.P. (1982). *Disruptive Pupils in Schools and Units.* Chichester: John Wiley & Sons.

Thomas, W.I. (1972). The definition of the situation. In J. Manis & A. Meltzer (Eds.), *Symbolic interaction* (pp. 331-336). Boston: Allyn & Bacon.

Tyler, W. (1988). *School organization: A sociological perspective.* London: Croom Helm.

VanderVen, K. (1991). Residential care, education, and treatment in the United States. In M. Gottesmann (Ed.), *Residential care: An international reader.* London: Whiting & Birch.

Waaldijk, K. (1994). The residential care worker. In M. Gottesmann (Ed.), *Recent changes and new trends in extrafamilial child care: An international perspective.* London; Whiting & Birch.

Walcoford, J. (1969). *The cloistered elite: A sociological analysis of the English public boarding school.* London: Macmillan.

Walker, B., & Gordon, J. (1977). Humor in the classroom. In P. Woods and M. Hammersley (Eds.), *School experience: Explorations in the sociology of education.* London: Croom Helm.

Weiner, A. (1991). Providing a development-enhancing environment: The child and youth care worker as observer and interpreter of behavior. In J. Beker & Z. Eisikovits (Eds.), *Knowledge utilization in residential child and youth care practice.* Washington, DC: Child Welfare League of America.

Werthman, C. (1963). Delinquents in school. *Berkeley Journal of Sociology, 8*(1), 39-60.

Wolins, M. (1969). Group care: Friend or foe? *Social Work,* 14(1), 35-53. (Also in M. Wolins (Ed.), *Successful group care: Explorations in the powerful environment.* Chicago: Aldine, 1974.)

Woods, P. (1976). Having a laugh: An antidote to schooling. In M. Hammersley & P. Woods (Eds.), *The process of schooling.* London: Routledge & Kegan Paul.

Woods, P. (1979). *The divided school.* London: Routledge & Kegan Paul.

Woods, P. (Ed.). (1980a). *Pupil strategies: Explorations in the sociology of the school.* London: Croom Helm.

Woods, P. (Ed.). (1980b). *Teacher strategies: Explorations in the sociology of the school.* London: Croom Helm.

Woods, P. (1981). Strategies, commitment, and identity: Making and breaking the teacher. In L. Barton & S. Walker (Eds.), *Schools, teachers, and teaching.* Lewes: Falmer.

Woods, P. (1983). Coping at school through humor. *British Journal of Sociology of Education, 4*(2), 111-124.

Woods, P. (1989). Stress and the teacher role. In M. Cole & S. Walker (Eds.), *Teaching and stress.* Milton Keynes: Open University Press.

Woods, P. (1990). *Teacher skills and strategies.* London: Falmer.

Woods, P., & Pollard, A. (Eds.). (1988). *Sociology and teaching.* London: Croom Helm.

Wozner, Y. (1991). Program integration in residential care: The residential center as the instrument of care delivery. In J. Beker & Z. Eisikovits (Eds.), *Knowledge utilization in residential child and youth care practice.* Washington, DC: Child Welfare League of America.

Appendix

The interviewees included 37 residential care workers in 14 coeducational residential care settings: nine youth villages (i.e., residential schools) and five care settings for youth from more problematic backgrounds who attend regular or special schools in the locality of the setting. Of the 37, 23 were men aged 22 to 38, all working as "madrichim" (plural of madrich). The 14 women interviewees were aged between 23 and 54, seven of them working as madrichas and 7 as "em-bayits" (housemothers). (A discussion of these roles appears in Chapter 1.)

MALE RESIDENTIAL CARE WORKERS

1. *Asher* worked for two years in a youth village, mostly with 16-17 year olds. He had a secondary school education and short-term in-service training courses for residential care workers. Three months after the interview he left the setting and the residential care field.

2. *Benny* has worked for ten years in a youth village; he has had considerable experience with youth in the three top classes in secondary school. He is a part-time undergraduate student at the university. He said that he had not wanted to be interviewed by me but agreed to do so to please his wife, an em-bayit who "for some reason thinks it's important for the kids."

3. *Dan* has worked in a youth village for four years. He is studying for a master's degree in the social sciences. Aged 35, he is older than the average madrich, a bachelor living alone in staff accommodations in the youth village. He sometimes writes in the local newspaper on education and social welfare. He asked for feedback and evaluation of his interview and didn't really believe there was no element of evaluation in the interview. "Are you telling me you don't represent the management in some way? Can this really be true?"

---

4. *Ephraim* has worked in a child care setting for just a year and a half. He is a student of business administration–quite a rare subject among care and education workers.

5. *Felix* has worked in residential care settings for eight years. He has a secondary school education and has taken short-term in-service training courses in residential care. At his initiative, the interview extended over two half-day sessions.

6. *Gad* has worked in a youth village for three years, mostly with the younger age groups. He has a degree in education. At the beginning of the interview he was demonstratively impatient; after seven minutes, he said, "Well, is there anything else you want to know?" His impatience disconcerted me; I thought the interview was lost, but after a while we both calmed down and in the end we spent almost four hours talking. On leaving he said, "I thought all this stuff was academic nonsense. To tell you the truth I still don't see how these discussions can help the kids, but maybe there's something in it. At least they do something for one's ego."

7. *Henry* has worked in a care setting for four years. He has a secondary school education and has taken short-term in-service training courses for residential care workers. He stressed several times in the course of the interview that this was the first time anybody had spoken with him about his work. He had always wanted to talk about it, but either there was no one to talk to or he was afraid.

8. *Isaac* has worked in a care setting for four years and had been one of my students.

9. *Jacob,* a youth village madrich with four years of experience, specialized in the intermediate ages (grades 9 and 10). He is a part-time undergraduate student at a teacher training college. He said, "The problem is not what happens between the madrich and his charges. The problem is that there are no firm rules on how to treat them and the madrich doesn't really know what's good for them. So he often feels guilty, thinking he may have unintentionally been unfair to them."

10. *Kedem* has had five years of experience working in a youth village, mostly with youth in the junior high school age range (grades 7, 8, and 9). He had a secondary school education and has taken short-term in-service training courses for residential care workers.

11. *Ken* works in a youth village with grades 9 and 10. He had been a student of mine in a master's degree program. During the interview he murmured a few times, half-seriously, half joking, "I do this work only because I don't have a stall in the market. Why the hell don't I have a stall in the market . . . ?"

12. *Leor* works with the senior class (aged 17) in a youth village. He is

a qualified teacher but says openly that he does not intend to go on working in education and social welfare. He plans to move into the diplomatic service as a junior attache or something similar. His family is of Middle Eastern origin but, nevertheless, he insisted repeatedly that the difference between Occidental and Mediterranean Jews is not cultural but genetic. "All that talk about equal ability is political, aimed to reassure. It doesn't help. It creates harmful illusions." He is devoted to his charges but shows no great faith in their ability to change.

13. *Mansur* has worked in a youth village for four years. He is studying social work.

14. *Naphtali* has worked for ten years in a care setting for children diagnosed as having severe psychological disturbances.

15. *Ohad* is a new madrich working in the same setting as Naphtali

16. *Porat* has been a youth village madrich for four years, and he is studying for a bachelor's degree in informal education.

17. *Reuben* has worked for three years in the same youth village as Porat.

18. *Shamoon* is a Christian Arab (the only interviewee who does not belong to the Jewish majority in Israel). (Educational occupations carry more prestige among Israeli Arabs than in the Jewish sector.) He says that he intends to work in residential care until he retires, and he hopes to be appointed principal of the setting shortly. He claims that discipline in educational settings in the Arab sector, certainly in his Church institution, is stricter than in the Jewish sector. He believes that many of the ills of Israeli society could be cured by strengthening discipline among the youth.

19. *Tal,* in his second year working in a youth village, has an unusually broad education. He is a top student who is working on his master's degree in the humanities and plans to continue for a third degree and a university career. He stood out among the interviewees for his belief in the youths' ability to change and his feeling that their dropping out from academic secondary schools was due to social circumstances, not poor ability. He hopes to teach in an academic secondary school for disadvantaged youth as well as at a university.

20. *Vardi* is in his third year working in a youth village. He excels in running music groups and vocal groups but is "not interested" in the "psychological and educational sides" of the madrich's work. In his opinion, his superiors place exaggerated stress on this "impractical" aspect of the work.

21. *Uzzi* is in his second year at a youth village. He and his wife work in the setting because it provides them with accommodations and other ser-

vices. They both work as madrichim, not out of a "sense of vocation," but because it is a convenient solution for a few years. His wife is pregnant with their first child and he is worried because their apartment is too small and there is no room for a baby. His wife will also have to reduce her working hours. He is afraid that their employers will think that it is not worth keeping them on in the setting. He likes the young people, "but not as a career."

22. *Yehuda* is in his third year at a youth village. In his spare time he is trying—with the knowledge of his employers—to develop a small business.

23. *Zvika* is in his third year working in a care setting.

FEMALE RESIDENTIAL CARE WORKERS

24. *Abigail,* who has been a madricha for three years, is very involved with her colleagues' rights and working conditions. She is studying for a master's degree in education.

25. *Batya* is a housemother in a youth village who had a secondary school education and has taken short-term in-service training courses for residential care workers. She wears "weird" clothes. At the beginning of the interview, she sat chewing gum with her mouth wide open, eyeing the interviewer with hostility. In the course of the conversation, she softened and even apologized: "I'm sorry I'm not dressed suitably. Sometimes I find that a bit hard. I really hope it doesn't offend you."

26. *Claire* was the most veteran residential care worker among those interviewed. She has worked for 22 years as an em-bayit, many of them as head em-bayit. To her, "The setting is home; the kids and the staff are family."

27. *Daniella* is a madricha in her third year at a youth village. She has a bachelor's degree in informal social education.

28. *Esther* has been a madricha in a care setting for two years and is about to graduate from a teacher training college. She decided to work in the setting after her divorce, in part to solve her financial problems and to establish a framework for her 11-year-old son.

29. *Flora* is a housemother in a care setting. She is a part-time undergraduate university student.

30. *Gretel,* a new housemother in a care setting, is a university graduate.

31. *Hilla* is a new housemother at a youth village. Born in the United States, she speaks Hebrew very well but every now and then slips into English replete with slang. She says that her main problem in life is the transition to a different culture. "With American kids, Jews or gentiles, I would get on better." She wants to get a master's degree in clinical

psychology, become a psychoanalyst, and apply to join the Israeli Psycho-analytical Institute. She thinks that as a group care worker she will never earn enough money and, more importantly, she will never really under-stand her charges' psychology.

32. *Ilana* has worked as a madricha in a care setting for three years.

33. *Judy* has been working for two years as a madricha in a care setting. She is studying for a bachelors degree in Psychology.

34. *Kalia* is in her seventh year as an em-bayit in a youth village.

35. *Leah,* a madricha in a youth village, had a secondary school educa-tion and has taken short-term in-service training courses for residential care workers.

36. *Mirit* began working as a madricha in a care setting six months before the interview.

37. *Nira* is a madricha in a care setting. She had a secondary school education and has taken short-term in-service training courses for residen-tial care workers. She is the focus of much social activity among her colleagues at the setting. The younger ones, especially, often drop by her apartment after work. Nira is a relative of a well-known political figure in Israeli society and thinks her colleagues suspect her of receiving special privileges. "But that's nonsense. It's very annoying when the people you work with say you have advantages you don't have. But they're all sure of it and it's no use trying to convince them it's not true. They would never believe me."

Index

action, 1,4-7,9,25-26,65,67,71,73,
76-77,81,83,85,92-93,
96-97,101,104
Adler. H., 22,107
affective, 33-37
ambivalent, 37,49
American, 107
Anglin, J. P., 22,107
Arieli, M., 9,12,22,45,93,98,105,
107,109 110,112
"avant-garde," 98-99

Ball, B. J., 9,51,107
bargaining, 13,77,88-92
Bar-Tal, D., 71,112
Becker, H. S., 100,106-107
Beker, J., 22,44,107-110,113-114
Beynon, J., 51,108
blame
downward displacement of,
34-35,44
upward displacement of, 39-40
Blase, J., 9,108
Bloome, D., 96,108
boarding schools, 15,108,110,113
Britain, 105
British mandate on Palestine, 97
Buber, M., 5,108
Bullock, R., 22,45,61,76,93,106,
108,111
burn-out, 4

Canada, 22,107
career, 2-3,96,101,103,106,109,
112,118
caring, 3,5,15,21

Carlebach, J., 16,108
Central Bureau of Statistics, Israel,
108
charisma, 77-78,80,86,91-92
Cherrett, P., 93,111
choice, 6,65,73,81,100,102,112
cognitive, 33-34
cognitive dissonance, 101,109
Cole, M., 9,108 109,111,114
Colla-Müller, H., 22,108
colleagues, 77,84-86,88-89,92,105
Collins, R., 39,108
Colton, M. J., 22,108
commitment, 9,13,49,95,97,
99-101,106-107,111,113
compliance
internalized, 61
strategic, 61,63
Comstock, D., 31,108
conflict, 3,9,19,21-22,27,76,100,
101,108-109,112
consensus 75,89
contentment, 2-3,9,95-96,103-105
Control, 51,57,71-72,75-78,80-81,
84-85,87-93,97,103,10-111
Cookson, P. W., 105,107
cooperation, 6,24-25,30-31,63-65,
73,75-81,83-85,87-89,
92-93,96
cooptation, 25,30-31,80,81-82,93
coping, 2,4,9,60,71,97,105
cosmopolitans, 16-18,110
countertransference, 102
course of action, 25,71,92
cultural
background, 3,36
boundaries, 9

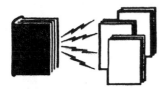

Haworth
DOCUMENT DELIVERY
SERVICE

This valuable service provides a single-article order form for any article from a Haworth journal.

- *Time Saving:* No running around from library to library to find a specific article.
- *Cost Effective:* All costs are kept down to a minimum.
- *Fast Delivery:* Choose from several options, including same-day FAX.
- *No Copyright Hassles:* You will be supplied by the original publisher.
- *Easy Payment:* Choose from several easy payment methods.

Open Accounts Welcome for . . .
- Library Interlibrary Loan Departments
- Library Network/Consortia Wishing to Provide Single-Article Services
- Indexing/Abstracting Services with Single Article Provision Services
- Document Provision Brokers and Freelance Information Service Providers

---

MAIL or *FAX* THIS ENTIRE ORDER FORM TO:

Haworth Document Delivery Service
The Haworth Press, Inc.
10 Alice Street
Binghamton, NY 13904-1580

or FAX: 1-800-895-0582
or CALL: 1-800-342-9678
9am-5pm EST

PLEASE SEND ME PHOTOCOPIES OF THE FOLLOWING SINGLE ARTICLES:

1) Journal Title: _____

   Vol/Issue/Year: _____ Starting & Ending Pages: _____

Article Title: _____

_____

2) Journal Title: _____

   Vol/Issue/Year: _____ Starting & Ending Pages: _____

Article Title: _____

_____

3) Journal Title: _____

   Vol/Issue/Year: _____ Starting & Ending Pages: _____

Article Title: _____

_____

4) Journal Title: _____

   Vol/Issue/Year: _____ Starting & Ending Pages: _____

Article Title: _____

(See other side for Costs and Payment Information)

COSTS: Please figure your cost to order quality copies of an article.

1. Set-up charge per article: $8.00
   ($8.00 × number of separate articles) _____

2. Photocopying charge for each article:

   1-10 pages: $1.00 _____

   11-19 pages: $3.00 _____

   20-29 pages: $5.00 _____

   30+ pages: $2.00/10 pages _____

3. Flexicover (optional): $2.00/article _____

4. Postage & Handling: US: $1.00 for the first article/
   $.50 each additional article _____

   Federal Express: $25.00 _____

   Outside US: $2.00 for first article/
   $.50 each additional article _____

5. Same-day FAX service: $.35 per page _____

   GRAND TOTAL: _____

METHOD OF PAYMENT: (please check one)

❏ Check enclosed ❏ Please ship and bill. PO # _____
   (sorry we can ship and bill to bookstores only! All others must pre-pay)

❏ Charge to my credit card: ❏ Visa; ❏ MasterCard; ❏ Discover;
   ❏ American Express;

Account Number: _____ Expiration date: _____

Signature: X _____

Name: _____ Institution: _____

Address: _____

_____

City: _____ State: _____ Zip: _____

Phone Number: _____ FAX Number: _____

MAIL or *FAX* THIS ENTIRE ORDER FORM TO:

Haworth Document Delivery Service	**or FAX:** 1-800-895-0582
The Haworth Press, Inc.	**or CALL:** 1-800-342-9678
10 Alice Street	9am-5pm EST)
Binghamton, NY 13904-1580	